1.25

600
Health

PAIN-FREE

LUKE BUCCI, Ph.D.

Pain
Free

The Definitive Guide to Healing Arthritis, Low-Back Pain, and Sports Injuries through Nutrition and Supplements

THE SUMMIT GROUP ❧ FORT WORTH, TEXAS

THE SUMMIT GROUP
1227 West Magnolia, Suite 500 • Fort Worth, Texas 76102

Printed in the United States of America.

96 97 98 99 010 6 5 4 3

Library of Congress Cataloging-in-Publication Data

Bucci, Luke.
    Pain-free : the definitive guide to healing arthritis, low-back pain, and sports injuries through nutrition and supplements / Luke Bucci.
        p. cm.
    Includes bibliographical references and index.
    ISBN 1-56530-161-7
    1. Arthritis–Diseases–Diet therapy. 2. Arthritis–Nutritional aspects. 3. Joints–Diseases–Diet therapy. 4. Joints–Wounds and injuries–Diet therapy. I. Title.
RC933.B83 1995
616.7'220654–dc20   94-47120
                                                                          CIP

ↄ

Jacket and book design by David Sims

ↄ

Jacket and book design by David Sims

Table of Contents

Tables

Foreword

As an osteopathic physician in practice for nearly thirty years now, I have always had a keen interest in the body's ability to regulate and heal itself, especially in relation to the dynamics of the musculoskeletal system. This sense of interest has never wavered.

I was in general practice for four years. I spent eight years running an emergency room at night, and twelve years teaching osteopathic manipulation and philosophy at the home of osteopathy (Kirksville, Missouri) while at the same time overseeing a practice that involved caring for post-trauma and chronic musculoskeletal dysfunctions. Then came three years of intensive work in a prominent Midwest spine rehabilitation center and, finally, a private practice of my own. Today, I devote my efforts to better understanding and caring for the chronic musculoskeletal problems associated with living.

One of my great frustrations is identifying and correcting a dysfunction, only to have that dysfunction return. The usual reason for this is the poor capacity of connective tissue to regenerate itself. This is because of wear and tear, injury, and the forces of gravity. Because of this, I became involved in "prolotherapy" (also known as sclerotherapy or reconstructive therapy) a number of years ago. In prolotherapy, I found a way to stimulate growth of tissue to tighten ligaments and restore some degree of continuity to joint regions. However, some frustration for me still remained. In some individuals, the quality of their tissues did not lend itself to regeneration, as some more healthier tissues would.

I had tried different vitamin and mineral supplements on patients. While I would get some degree of help with this method, it was not always totally satisfactory. During this time, I found the much advertised and much used nonsteroidal anti-inflammatory drugs (NSAIDs) to be not only totally inadequate, but indeed detrimental to the healing process.

In recent years, I had also experienced increasing problems with my own back. These problems included degenerative changes, gradual destruction of cartilage, and the effects of aging combined with gravitational strain.

About a year and a half ago, at the suggestion of a colleague, I began taking a nutraceutical containing glucosamine, manganese ascorbate, and chondroitin sulfates. It worked. In a few short months, I began to feel relief from my chronic, nagging musculoskeletal pain. By the end of three months, I could honestly say that I had improved by some 90 percent.

Since then, I have gone on to use this product in my practice. To date, I have hundreds of satisfied patients who have switched from products that promise relief but do not help the overall healing of the body, to something that gives relief by allowing and assisting the body to heal itself.

I wish everyone could experience this. Unfortunately, it is an uphill climb to get this information out to the general public. We have a lot of information—much of it conflicting and/or confusing—flooding our systems every day, presented very effectively by drug companies and many physicians. Thankfully, we also have a scientist and author such as Dr. Luke Bucci whose devotion and attention have brought about this book. I hope it will inform the public of what might seem like a new concept. Frankly, in my case, this concept is as old as osteopathy.

Read and ingest this information. Present it to your physician. See if you can generate an interest in helping to heal and maintain your body through its own mechanisms, rather than looking for transient relief through drugs.

I would caution you that it takes time and perseverance in taking any nutraceutical. We live in an age of instant gratification, where it is believed that if something doesn't work within a few hours or days, we toss it aside. You must be willing to commit yourself to a few months' use, and commit yourself to taking on the responsibility of improving your lifestyle to enhance the ability of your body to heal itself. I certainly hope you enjoy the information you are given, and take it to heart. Then you, too, will want to thank Dr. Bucci.

Larry W. Bader, D.O.
Columbia, Missouri

Preface

Arthritis is the number-one disability in the United States. Yet, there's no medical cure and none in sight.

Joint disorders such as arthritis aren't fatal; therefore, they attract little media coverage. There exists minimal scientific research interest in joint health, at least when compared to heart disease, cancer, and AIDS. This lack of real concern is particularly frustrating for the many millions of arthritis sufferers, as well as their physicians, who have to treat their patients with less-than-ideal methods. Doctors and health-care professionals specializing in joint problems deserve kudos for the wonderful job they are doing with limited weapons. They fight a war limited in ways that suggest a modern-day soldier trying to survive on the battlefield armed only with a dueling pistol.

Help is on the way, however. And it's closer than many realize. As a researcher and clinical nutritionist, I've been able to uncover an enormous amount of medical information detailing the role simple nutrients play in healing joints. But somehow, this information has *not* been utilized in America, despite the fact that some of these nutrients *now* are the drugs of choice for the treatment of osteoarthritis in several European countries.

Amazingly, American doctors and researchers are almost completely ignorant of these very helpful, simple, and relatively inexpensive nutrients. It's time you learned about these life-enhancing measures for arthritis sufferers.

One of my lifelong commitments has been to educate physicians on the value of "clinical nutrition"—the use of nutrients in clinical settings. When I teach relicensing seminars or give educational presentations to physicians, they are shocked. Their skepticism centers around the traditional belief that nutrients can't actually help joint health. I say nutrients can help because I know it to be true. I don't make up this stuff. It's there in black and white for all the world to see, if you know where to look.

Look no further. It's all in here.

Being a thorough investigator (maybe even compulsive), I dug deeper and deeper into the medical journals at the Texas Medical Center Library in Houston, Texas. Over time I came across so much fascinating and corroborating information, that I knew it would take a book—this book—to get all the information out to the needing-to-know public.

Obviously, I can't educate *all* physicians in one lifetime, but I figured I could at least start reeducating many of these physicians by offering a comprehensive nutrition/joint healing book published by a reputable and prestigious scientific publisher. That turned out to be CRC Press in Boca Raton, Florida, which published my book, *Nutrition Applied to Injury Rehabilitation and Sports Medicine.* Whereas that first work is a scientific book on the topic of nutrition and joint healing to reach doctors and researchers, this book is tailored for general consumption. *Pain-Free* is necessary to reach as many people as possible—and tell them the good news about joint conditions, regardless of whether the condition is arthritis or an injury.

You don't have to wade through many boring technical explanations in this book to learn how to use nutrients to improve joint health. Also, I relate real-life experiences about these nutrients—information not suitable for scientific books. This brings the message home to you and me. After reading about these wonderful nutrients and seeing some of the results in my family, friends, and pets, I knew it was time to educate everyone. My goal is to inform you about your joints, and what you can do to help your joints help themselves.

Keep in mind that the application of nutrients for joint health is *not* intended to replace your current medical diagnosis and treatments. Instead, using nutrients for joint health should be a complement and an aid to whatever else you and your doctor are doing. It would be a serious mistake to rely solely upon nutrients without working closely with your doctor.

This brings up another point: Nutrients are not drugs. Although you might be taking pills that look like drugs, nutrients act in a completely different manner than most drugs. Some nutrients with health benefits are called "nutraceuticals." Nutraceuticals are what the body wants and can utilize normally. But drugs act differently. For this reason, nutrients and drugs *can* coexist. After all, you continue to eat if you are on medication, right? This book simply shows you how to target your nutrient intake to focus on joint health. My goal is to give your joints what they are hungry for. In turn, your joints can help themselves to their best possible extent. Drugs and medical treatments should also be able to assist your body in its healing response.

Let's face it, health is precious. Our bodies are constantly trying to be healthy, but we and our environment keep making that attempt difficult. Nutrition is but one way to support your body in doing what comes naturally—healing.

Remember that anything, nutrition included, is not a cure-all or panacea. Each person is unique and different. Therefore, interpret the results presented in this book with caution. You might or might not achieve what others have done. No matter what happens, you at least have made your body healthier. Hopefully, your attempts will be enough to make a real difference in the health of your joints.

Most likely, the information in this book will be relatively new to you. Take your time, reflect, digest, act, and, most of all, enjoy the information.

Luke R. Bucci, Ph.D., C.C.N., C.(A.S.C.P.), C.N.S.
Houston, Texas

Acknowledgments

Any book is a joint effort by the author and many other people. I would like to extend thanks to the many people who have helped shape my life and who have offered support throughout the writing of this book.

First, my wife Naniece deserves tremendous praise for putting up with a husband who was using up air, food, and clothes, but had little time to interact. She has truly been marvelous.

My family also needs to be included, particularly my father, Robert Joseph Francis Bucci, M.D., for arousing my curiosity about the human body. Watching all those autopsies has really been impressive.

I would like to thank University of Houston professor Ira Wolinsky, Ph.D., for being my series editor for the CRC Press, as well as Harvey Kane and his staff at the CRC Press. They had the wisdom and foresight to publish the first scientific book on application of nutrients for musculoskeletal healing.

The staff at SpectraCell Laboratories (my day job) has also been very supportive in putting up with me on those frantic days. Other peers and colleagues deserve mention, and I deeply apologize if I have left anyone out. Thanks to (in alphabetical order):

Karen Jo Briggs, Dr. Susan Brown, Dr. Michael Colgan, Paul DeVerter III, Esq., Dr. Alan Gaby, Dr. Charles Gasaway, Dr. Ann Grandjean, Dr. Jim Heffley, Winna Henry, Dr. Jim Hickson, Dr. Russell Jaffe, Dr. Phil Kaufmann, Dr. William Kaufman, Dr. Jerry Koch, Dr. Marvin Meistrich, Dr. Michael Murray, Dr. Gary Osborn, Dr. Henk Oswald, Dr. Cleve Phillips, Dr. Kenneth Rennie, Jarrow Rogovin, Dr. Michael Schmidt, Cliff Sheats, Dr. Elizabeth Travis, Dr. Dave Watts, and others for their thoughtful discussions.

A special thanks goes to Dr. Robert Henderson for providing contacts with real people who are using nutrients to help their joints, along with those who graciously shared their stories to enlighten this book.

Dr. Larry Bader deserves special mention for his foreword. He is in the medical trenches, using nutrients along with other medical methods to assist those with joint problems. His wisdom is real-life.

Of course, I would like to thank the wonderful staff at The Summit Group, especially Len Oszustowicz, Mike Towle, and Maggie Greenwood-Robinson, for really making this book possible. They have shown wisdom and foresight in publishing a book that will help many people.

Finally, I thank you, the reader, for being interested in your health. Good luck!

How to Use This Book

Nearly all the information in this book was obtained from reputable scientific sources. Only the latest (since 1990) medical textbooks were used as sources for information on what arthritis is, the treatments, joint injuries, and nutrition. The information on nutrients is found in many individual scientific journal articles. Peer-reviewed articles (meaning of the highest scientific caliber) have been used 99 percent of the time.

The only information not found in authoritative texts or scientific articles are individual case reports and unpublished data that I have accumulated during ten years of working in the field of nutrition. This amounts to insider information and will always be ahead of scholarly writings. Twenty years from now, all this information will probably be in medical textbooks.

Sources for each chapter are included in the back of the book under the heading "References" and listed in alphabetical order by the first author's name. For the sake of reading simplicity, reference numbers or footnotes aren't included within the text. Often, specific articles are mentioned in the text. The whole point is to inform you that there is a considerable amount of good science behind the use of nutrients for treating joint conditions.

Of course, you are encouraged to seek out any of these sources to supplement your knowledge of joint problems in specific areas.

If you need further scientific documentation, you may contact the CRC Press in Boca Raton, Florida (800-272-7737) for a copy of my scientific book titled *Nutrition Applied to Injury Rehabilitation and Sports Medicine*, published in November 1994. This book covers the topic of nutrition and healing of injuries, arthritis, surgical wounds, and other musculoskeletal injuries in a thorough, scholarly fashion. This book is not for the faint-hearted, as it contains 1,381 reference sources. Thus, there's ample scientific evidence for the information in this book. The conventional scientific background of the author, combined with using (almost exclusively) reputable scientific sources, makes the information in this book beyond reproach.

Parts of your body that you might be unfamiliar with are described in chapter two. A glossary at the end of the book has been included to help you understand new names and learn what your body is doing.

This book will help you use to your advantage the latest information on specific nutrients that can benefit degenerative joint disease, low-back pain, joint injuries, and many other joint conditions. You'll learn what these nutrients are, where to get them, how to use them, and what to expect, depending upon your condition. You'll also be able to learn more about what your joints are, and how they can go wrong. But the bottom line is that finally there's good news for those suffering from osteoarthritis and other degenerative joint conditions. You can do something positive!

PART ONE

The Pain
That
Comes
and
Goes

1

What Kind of Arthritis Do You Have?

The pain in your back comes and goes. Sometimes it's so stiff you can hardly move. Other times, it just aches with a dull throb.

Are these just the aches and pains of old age? Not necessarily.

You might be among the millions suffering from arthritis, a serious and potentially crippling disease. Arthritis attacks the joints, as well as the muscle and connective tissue surrounding them. To make matters worse, there are more than one hundred different forms of arthritis. It can be caused by injuries, a weakened immune system, wear and tear on the joints, infections, or genetic factors. Unless you've seen a doctor for an accurate diagnosis, there's no telling what kind you have.

Here's something you probably didn't realize: Arthritis and other diseases of the musculoskeletal system are the number-one medical problem in the world. They are bigger than cancer, heart disease, and AIDS. Unlike those diseases, however, musculoskeletal problems are rarely fatal. That's why there's little media attention focused on them. On top of that, research to find cures is greatly underfunded. Arthritis is practically ignored because of the old squeaky-wheel axiom, or in this case, creaky joint.

It's no wonder the musculoskeletal system breaks down. After all, it's much like a machine, complete with movable, mechanical parts. But machine parts wear out, give way, even fail altogether. You know this from owning and operating appliances and cars. So do our bodies. Think of how much motion and physical stress your body is subjected to day in and day out. It's a machine that runs around the clock. But unlike machines, broken-down bodies *can* repair themselves. Musculoskeletal problems *can* be fixed.

MANY DIFFERENT ARTHRITIS DISEASES

■ The term *arthritis* literally means "inflamed joints," taken from the Greek words *arthron* (joint) and *itis* (inflammation). Of the one hundred different forms of the disease, following is a rundown of the more common:

Osteoarthritis (OA). This also is known as degenerative joint disease—osteoarthritis that takes place as you age. Joint tissue deteriorates, and cartilage, a protective padding around bones, begins to break down.

The most notable sign of osteoarthritis is a dull, aching feeling in a joint. The most commonly affected areas of the body include the spine, hip, knees, neck, hands, fingers, and feet. This book focuses primarily on osteoarthritis, which is the most common cause of pain and physical handicaps among older people throughout the world. Most physicians will tell you that osteoarthritis is usually not reversible. But it can be, as will be explained.

Rheumatoid Arthritis (RA). This form of arthritis is thought to be a disease whereby the body's immune system attacks itself. It strikes people of all ages. More than two million people in America have it. Most are women.

Symptoms include fever, fatigue, muscle weakness, loss of appetite, and depression. Joints feel stiff, especially in the morning, although the stiffness improves with activity. Around affected joints, there is usually swelling, nodules (small lumps), limited movement, and pain. Rheumatoid arthritis is "symmetrical," too, occurring in the same joint on both sides of the body.

RA can lead to joint deformity and crippling—when people hear about the horrors of "arthritis," RA is the usual culprit. Because of the crippling potential, RA has attracted much more research and popular attention than has osteoarthritis.

Juvenile Rheumatoid Arthritis. This affects children under age sixteen. It is characterized by stiff, swollen joints that are filled with fluid. These symptoms last longer than six weeks. Other symptoms include fever and enlarged lymph nodes, spleen, and liver. Frequently, there's also inflammation of the eyes. In young children, there might be abnormal bone growth, and later in life, bone thinning. Twenty percent of children with this form of arthritis will continue to deteriorate. Many side effects are caused by the powerful drugs used to reduce symptoms.

Seronegative Polyarthritis. This is a milder form of rheumatoid arthritis, one that's less crippling. People with seronegative polyarthritis have a better chance for improvement than those with rheumatoid arthritis.

Ankylosing Spondylitis (AS). Usually starting at age twenty, ankylosing spondylitis affects joints of the trunk, including the pelvis and spine. Over time, the spine gradually stiffens. The good news is that only 20 percent of those with AS become disabled twenty years after diagnosis.

Other symptoms include pain, stiffness, inability to expand the chest, and often eye inflammation.

AS is a cause of low-back pain that persists for more than three months. Rest doesn't seem to help, but exercise does. AS-related low-back pain can hurt so much that it forces sufferers out of bed at night.

Reiter's Syndrome (RS). This form of arthritis strikes men primarily, especially sailors or soldiers with a recent case of diarrhea or dysentery. Christopher Columbus was disabled by RS-like symptoms. He died at age fifty-five, crippled by arthritis.

About 2 percent of people infected by an epidemic of diarrhea will get Reiter's Syndrome. It usually affects the toes, feet, ankles, and knees first. There is inflammation of connective tissue that causes pain in the joints. With time, Reiter's Syndrome can look like rheumatoid arthritis and lead to permanent joint damage.

Psoriatic Arthritis (PSA). About one in ten people with psoriasis (a skin condition) will develop psoriatic arthritis. It usually starts about ten to twenty years after psoriasis begins. PSA tends to be inherited. It is characterized by pitting of fingernails, some type of spinal arthritis, and erosion of the outermost finger joints. There are no serious complications or loss of function. Five percent of PSA sufferers, however, will develop hand deformities.

Enteropathic Arthritis. This is a form of "reactive arthritis," so named because certain types of inflammatory bowel diseases trigger the immune system to attack joints. Crohn's disease, ulcerative colitis, celiac disease, and intestinal bypass surgery for obesity are among the illnesses associated with inflammatory arthritis.

Outer joints—those of the toes, feet, ankles, hands, and fingers—show arthritis most often. A type of inflammatory arthritis can affect the hips and spine as well. Enteropathic arthritis subsides in about six weeks.

Infectious Arthritis. This is the name given to joint inflammation caused by parasites, viruses, fungi, and other microbes. The microbe enters the body through the bloodstream and travels to the joint, causing arthritis-like symptoms.

Lyme Disease. This illness gets its name from the Lyme region in Connecticut, where in 1975 some children showed symptoms of arthritis, including an initial skin rash. The cause of the disease was eventually traced to deer ticks infected with a new strain of bacteria. Between three and thirty-two days after being bitten, a person gets a skin rash. The bacteria then invades the bloodstream and travels to other tissues. Some weeks later, there is pain and stiffness in the joints, as well as other problems affecting the skin and central nervous system. The symptoms are very similar to those of rheumatoid arthritis.

As of late summer 1994, about twenty thousand people in the United States had Lyme Disease. New laboratory tests have made its diagnosis more accurate than ever before.

Bacterial Arthritis. This is an infection of the joint or nearby bone. Although it can occur in any age group, bacterial arthritis strikes people with suppressed immune systems, joint replacement patients, the elderly, children, intravenous drug users, HIV-infected individuals, and rheumatoid arthritis patients taking certain medications. Parasites found in the tropics are often the culprits behind the infection.

Bacterial arthritis comes on suddenly, usually affecting one joint. The joint becomes warm, tender, and swollen with fluid. There might be high fever and chills as well. Unless treatment with antibiotics is begun early, there could be permanent damage to the joints.

Viral Arthritis. Arthritis can set in after a viral infection such as mumps, German measles, hepatitis B, and HIV. This has prompted some investigators to search for a link between viruses and rheumatoid arthritis. If caught and treated in time, viral arthritis is short-lived. Though rarely seen in the United States, untreated viral arthritis can lead to a slow but steady loss of joint function, as well as permanent disability.

OSTEOARTHRITIS
The Biggest Medical Problem in the World

■ Of all forms of arthritis, osteoarthritis is the most prevalent. Consider some staggering facts:

◆ More than 80 percent of people older than age fifty-five have osteoarthritis–this equates to about fifty-five million Americans.

◆ Approximately two out of three people age thirty-five and older have osteoarthritis.

◆ About 20 percent of the United States population has osteoarthritis, compared to less than 2 percent for rheumatoid arthritis. Osteoarthritis is a much bigger problem than rheumatoid arthritis by thirty to fifty times. Put another way: One out of five people has osteoarthritis; one out of one hundred has rheumatoid arthritis.

◆ In the U.S., there are three hundred thousand hip replacements, three hundred thousand low-back operations, and three hundred thousand knee replacements performed annually, mostly due to osteoarthritis.

◆ As many as 90 percent of us will get osteoarthritis at some point in our lives.

◆ Osteoarthritis is a worldwide problem, disabling people of all ages. (See Tables 1.1 and 1.2.)

When you add the equally staggering number of injuries to joints, every one of us could have some kind of joint problem sooner or later! Injuries regularly occur from sports, recreation, home, accidents, and work at alarming rates. In 1976, 7 percent of all doctor office visits were for chronic or acute injuries. Compare this figure to 11 percent of all office visits being for osteoarthritis and rheumatoid arthritis. This amounts to about one out of five doctor office visits caused by joints. You can therefore see that our joints are a major reason we hurt enough to go see a doctor.

Six Telltale Signs of Osteoarthritis

■ How do you know if you have osteoarthritis? Unfortunately, osteoarthritis isn't like other disorders that have clear-cut symptoms. It's as frustrating for your doctor to identify as it is for you. Knowing the signs, however, can prompt you to get early treatment—treatment that can help you avoid or reverse this potentially crippling condition.

There are six telltale signs:

1. Pain. Usually around joints, the pain is dull and aching. Its source is hard to pinpoint. In the early stages of osteoarthritis, the affected joints hurt most after you use them. Eventually, they also begin to ache while at rest. When joint degeneration is severe, the pain is so bad that it wakes you up at night. There's no doubt about it—osteoarthritis hurts.

There are no nerves in cartilage, so you might wonder how osteoarthritis can cause pain. Good question.

Although damaged, the cartilage itself isn't the source of pain. The pain stems from other joint structures, of which nerves are getting pinched, squeezed, or stretched beyond their limits. Two other sources of pain are inflammation and the swelling of veins in the bone underneath cartilage.

Pain is the most important symptom—one that prompts you to see your doctor. Unfortunately, by the time you feel pain, there's considerable joint damage. Cartilage repair then becomes more difficult.

2. **Stiffness.** Most people with osteoarthritis experience frozen or stiff joints most intensely in the morning or following exertion. The stiffness lasts for only fifteen to thirty minutes—unlike rheumatoid arthritis, where it lasts for hours. You've probably heard of people who can predict the weather by their "lumbago" (an arthritic condition in the low back). Don't laugh. It's well established that changes in weather can cause joint stiffness and pain.

> *Pain is the most important symptom—one that prompts you to see your doctor.*

3. **Crepitus.** This term describes joints that creak like a hinge in need of oil. Having a creaky joint doesn't mean you have osteoarthritis. Yet, if your joint is painful, stiff—and even creaky—then it's likely you do have osteoarthritis. Crepitus gets worse as osteoarthritis progresses.

4. **Joint Immobility.** The worse and more advanced your osteoarthritis, the harder it is to bend your knees, rotate your shoulder, or move your hips—depending on the joint involved. Joints can even give way without warning.

5. **Joint Changes.** Bony overgrowth around joints (osteophytes) or inflammation of the joint cavity lining (synovitis) can cause enlargement of a joint. Other joint changes include deformity and dislocation. These indicate a very advanced

stage of osteoarthritis in which cartilage is lost and the bone underneath the cartilage collapses. What's more, bony overgrowth can actually shove a bone out of joint. An example is bowleggedness, a result of knees badly damaged by osteoarthritis.

6. **Muscle Shrinkage.** Many people stop exercising or being active after experiencing joint pain. When muscles aren't used enough, they waste away. This disrupts joint mechanics, and might cause joints to give way.

Osteoarthritis from Head to Toe

■ The main characteristics of osteoarthritis are pain, stiffness, and immobility around almost any joint. Still, the disorder manifests itself differently in different joints. Osteoarthritis of the hand, for example, might produce a level of discomfort quite unlike that of osteoarthritis of the hip. What follows is a brief discussion of these joint-to-joint differences.

HANDS AND WRISTS

In some people with osteoarthritis of the hand, bony lumps (Heberden's nodes) form on the outermost finger joints. Another frequently reported symptom is the formation of cysts that flare up on the affected joints. Eventually, all the fingers become arthritic, and possibly deformed. This type of osteoarthritis is believed to be hereditary and occurs mostly in women over fifty.

Osteoarthritis can attack the middle finger joints as well, forming bony lumps (Bouchard's nodes). This tends to strike postmenopausal women with a genetic tendency toward the disorder.

Another form of the disorder that destroys finger joints is "erosive osteoarthritis." Its symptoms are similar to those of rheumatoid arthritis.

The joints connecting fingers to the hand are susceptible to osteoarthritis from trauma or disease. When these joints are severely damaged, it's difficult to grasp objects. Performing routine tasks such as writing or brushing teeth is very painful.

Men in their thirties often get a type of osteoarthritis called "carpal boss," which afflicts the joints connecting the hand to the wrist. Its chief symptom is a firm, tender mass on the back of the hand covering the affected joints. The joints gradually become arthritic in the wake of accidents, such as fractures or finger dislocations. Likewise, repetitive stresses, fractures, and injuries to the thumb can trigger osteoarthritis of this joint.

The wrist joint is an easy target for osteoarthritis. The major symptoms are pain in the wrist, swelling that ebbs and flows, stiffness, weakness, and snapping noises during movement. Osteoarthritis of the wrist at one time was treated by surgically inserting a silicone implant into the joint. But the "cure" was worse than the disorder. Inflammation would set in, destroying bones and joints. This surgical treatment quickly fell out of favor.

ELBOWS AND SHOULDERS

Osteoarthritis of the elbow has been diagnosed in 95 percent of all people over age fifteen. Fortunately, cartilage destruction is mild or insignificant in most cases. In more severe cases, osteoarthritis of the elbow is disabling. Eating, lifting objects, brushing your hair, even the simple turning of doorknobs can make life miserable. In osteoarthritis of the elbow, loose pieces of connective tissue often float around in the joint. If damage can't be controlled, the elbow joint might have to be replaced with an artificial joint.

Osteoarthritis of the shoulder is common. Sixty percent of all people older than age fifteen have it. As we age, more shoulder arthritis shows up, so that 80 percent of people older than fifty-five and 94 percent of people older than seventy-four have some shoulder arthritis. Shoulder dislocations and overhand motions that place unusual stress on the shoulder, such as weightlifting, baseball throwing, football throwing, or tennis serving, can lead to osteoarthritis of the shoulder in young or old people.

Shoulder problems are hard to diagnose because the shoulder joint is actually several joints all wrapped together. Nerve impingements, tendinitis, and injuries of the rotator cuff all increase the chances of getting osteoarthritis in the shoulder later in life. Like the elbow, the shoulder joint can be replaced with an artificial joint.

> *Shoulder problems are hard to diagnose because the shoulder joint is actually several joints all wrapped together.*

TEMPOROMANDIBULAR JOINT (TMJ OR JAW JOINT)

The TMJ of the jaw allows us to eat and talk because of its wide range of motion. Recently, TMJ Syndrome has become a condition popular to treat, although a clear, consensus definition doesn't yet exist. Usually, pain in the TMJ area is due to spasms of the chewing muscles. Pain is worst in the morning, and gets even worse when people are under emotional stress. Any age can be affected, but most commonly, women in their forties show these symptoms. TMJ Syndrome is not really degenerative joint disease, but it might cause imbalance in the TMJ that later leads to real osteoarthritis.

Unlike TMJ Syndrome, true osteoarthritis of the temporomandibular joint exhibits pain that gets worse as the day progresses. Pain is felt at the joint itself and usually not in the jaw muscle. Careful attention to diagnosis must be made because osteoarthritis of the TMJ can become chronic.

SPINE AND LOWER BACK

In the neighborhood of the spine, there are some two hundred separate joint surfaces, plus a complex network of nerves, ligaments, and other connective tissues. It's no wonder the spine is the most common target for osteoarthritis. The major causes of spinal osteoarthritis are aging, trauma, congenital (born-with) conditions, other joint diseases, and certain metabolic diseases.

The spine is divided into three sections: cervical (neck); thoracic (trunk); and lumbar (lower back). All can be attacked with full force by osteoarthritis.

Osteoarthritis in the neck is most often a result of injury or degeneration of the cervical spine. The injury compresses or squeezes the nerves there, causing pain. Whiplash from a car wreck does the same thing.

Osteoarthritis of the neck strikes people between the ages of twenty and fifty. One obvious symptom is pain; others include weakness or a loss of feeling in the shoulders, arms, hands, or fingers. Older people get more nerve compression in their necks from osteophytes (bony overgrowth). Blood vessels and nerves can also get compressed, leading to dizziness, vertigo, blurred vision, and headaches. These symptoms are a result of arteries in the head being squeezed, thus reducing blood flow to the brain. Usually, brain symptoms from spinal osteoarthritis come and go.

Osteoarthritis in the trunk is far less common than that of the neck and low back. It sets in after age thirty, as the spongy cushions (discs) between the vertebrae begin to degenerate. Parts of the discs dry out and become torn, eventually protruding (herniating) into areas where they don't belong. The body tries to patch up the damage by forming osteophytes. But this creates its own set of problems, namely nerve compression (squeezing). As a result, there's pain in the back, as well as in other parts of the body.

Osteoarthritis in the lower back can be caused by excessive use, injury, or the aging process. It is one of the many causes of low-back pain.

The cartilage discs separating vertebrae degenerate (become worn out), and the spaces between them grow narrow. Disc herniation can occur even when osteoarthritis is not yet severe. Osteophytes tend to form, altering joint loads and providing a barrier against further protrusion of the discs. However, osteophytes themselves can squeeze nerves, just like herniated discs. Symptoms include localized or radiating pain, tenderness, and stiffening of the back. The pain comes and goes before it becomes disabling. Usually, it hurts more to move. Lying down eases the pain.

Sciatica is a well-known stabbing or shooting pain that starts in the low back or buttock and shoots down a leg. People with sciatica may lean or list to one side. The classic situation of bending over and then not being able to straighten up is sciatica, which has been illustrated in many movies and television shows. There are several causes of sciatica, all of which involve pinching or squeezing a nerve root. Osteoarthritis of the spine is one possibility.

Spinal stenosis is another common form of low-back pain caused by degenerative joint conditions. Nerves or the spinal cord itself get pinched by bony overgrowth, leading to many vague symptoms such as pains, cramps, numbness, and tingling in the legs. When the spinal stenosis is really severe, people cannot sleep lying down; they have to sleep in a seated position.

HIP

The hip is the second most common joint affected by severe osteoarthritis, next to the spine. Injuries, osteoarthritis itself, and congenital abnormalities all speed up degeneration of the hip joint.

Sufferers variously describe their pain as deep, dull, aching, or boring. Pain is present at rest, at night, and during any weight-bearing activity. Burning or throbbing pain might indicate other joint problems such as rheumatoid arthritis. Osteoarthritis in the hip might produce pain in other nearby parts of the body.

When the pain is severe enough, your quality of life is affected. Walking, climbing stairs, dressing, and sleeping become difficult, painful activities. You might even start to limp while walking.

Although it can occur at any age, degenerative joint disease in the hip is most often seen in people over the age of sixty. Each year more than one hundred thousand Americans undergo reconstructive surgery of the hip.

KNEE

The third most common joint susceptible to osteoarthritis is the knee. The chief symptoms are pain during movement, and stiffness in the morning or after sitting. Interestingly, stiffness improves with activity, but gets worse later in the day. Other symptoms include physical locking of the joint, a clicking noise, or a grinding sound. Sometimes, there is swelling around the joint. Osteoarthritis in the knee is usually the result of an earlier injury or surgery in the knee joint. Over time, the affected joints cause bowleggedness or knock-knees.

ANKLES AND FEET

Osteoarthritis in these joints is less common than in knees or hips. The usual joint affected in the feet is the big toe. A knob forms on top of the joint. This makes walking difficult and uncomfortable. Deformity might later develop as the joint enlarges.

In any foot joint with osteoarthritis, pain always is worse in the morning and while walking. There's also accompanying warmth and swelling. Range of motion is limited. Walking to accommodate the affected joint can put strain on other joints, such as the knee.

With osteoarthritis in the ankle, most people can walk comfortably on flat surfaces. But walking on irregular or uneven surfaces causes pain, balance problems, and loss of agility. The foot might even begin to tilt. Limping is common.

People with osteoarthritis in the ankle report pain, swelling, and warmth around the joint. The pain forces them to walk in such a way that too much stress is placed on the knee.

Diagnosing Osteoarthritis

■ So, do you really have osteoarthritis? Certain physical evidence such as the symptoms described here will point to that possibility. But please don't self-diagnose. Only *your doctor* can tell for sure. Plus, your doctor might be able to put the brakes on osteoarthritis if detected early enough and treated correctly.

One way to identify joint damage is by an X-ray. This test is not always a reliable indicator, however. You might want to have an MRI (magnetic resonance imaging) performed. By using magnetism and radio waves, an MRI produces detailed pictures of the inside of the body. These pictures are transferred to film and enhanced by sophisticated computer technology. The exam is safe, painless, and noninvasive.

On the Outside Looking In

■ So far we've looked at various symptoms—those outer signs of osteoarthritis. But what's really going on in there?

During the early stages of osteoarthritis, the surfaces of cartilage start to fray like poorly woven cloth. Then they thicken and become waterlogged in the process. These biochemical changes alter the structure of the joints, further aggravating the osteoarthritis. Patches of cartilage start to unravel. The joints turn on their own cartilage, releasing destructive enzymes bent on demolishing it. With this demolition come tears in the cartilage. Pieces break off and start floating around in the joints. More cartilage is lost.

In the later stages of osteoarthritis, no cartilage is made. Without cartilage to cushion the joints, bones begin to grind on bones.

Deterring the Disease

■ There was a time—and it really wasn't that long ago—when scientists believed that cartilage was irreparable. In experiments, cartilage was cut, drilled, or sanded. Afterward, it showed no attempt to repair itself. As for any healing response, cartilage was chalked up as a lost cause. The only time cartilage appeared to mend itself was when it and its underlying bone were both damaged. Bleeding from the damaged bone formed a scar at the wound site. But like a patch on an inner tube, this scar tissue didn't have the same strength or resiliency of real cartilage.

> *Now we know that cartilage does indeed repair itself, although very slowly.*

Now we know that cartilage does indeed repair itself, although very slowly. The hard part is stimulating cartilage to heal. To do so, it needs an extra metabolic nudge.

Enter "chondroprotection" (KONN-droe-pro-TEK-shon). This simply means repairing damaged cartilage and preventing its breakdown. Chondroprotection is not a new concept. It has been studied for more than twenty-five years, mostly in Europe.

Much like light switches, substances called "chondroprotective agents" turn on the cartilage-fixing process. They also help lubricate the joints and improve circulation around them. Unlike some drugs, chondroprotective agents work *with* the body, not *against* it.

Several biochemical compounds found in our own bodies and naturally in our foods show tremendous promise as chondroprotective agents. They are not drugs; they are simple nutrients that help stimulate the often complex cartilage-repair process.

You'll learn about these nutrients in Part Two. But first, let's take a look at the parts of the body where these nutrients do their job of repair and rejuvenation.

Who Gets Osteoarthritis?

Age	Percentage of Population with Severe Osteoarthritis
0-15	less than 2 percent
15-24	0-4 percent (looking at hands and feet only)
15-44	2-3 percent
15 and up	20 percent
45-64	25-40 percent
65 and up	37-90 percent

NOTE: Severe osteoarthritis limits joint movement or causes people to seek treatment for pain.

TABLE 1.1

Osteoarthritis Worldwide

Group	Percentage of Population with Osteoarthritis
Alaskan Eskimos	24 percent
United States Caucasians	44 percent
South African Blacks	53 percent
Rural Jamaicans	62 percent
English	70 percent
Pima and Blackfoot Native Americans	74 percent

TABLE 1.2

2

What You Don't Know About Your Joints Can Hurt You

If you could see inside your musculoskeletal system, you would find a masterfully designed network of muscles, bones, and connective tissue. This system is the structural support for your body, giving you the ability to walk, run, jump, and move with amazing freedom. What's more, it protects your vital organs, with the ribs surrounding the delicate lungs and heart, and the skull encasing the brain. Let's go inside and watch this well-engineered system at work.

Those Movable Parts Called Joints

■ You probably never notice your joints, at least not until there's pain, stiffness, or some creaky-sounding noise. Joints are the structures where the ends of bones meet. There are three types of joints in the body, and the most common are the synovial joints. These make movement possible and operate much like hinges on a door or joysticks in a video game. The hinge of the knee and the ball and socket of the hip are examples of synovial joints.

The bone ends are cushioned with a padding of smooth elastic tissue (cartilage). The space inside the joints is filled with a small amount of lubricating fluid (synovial fluid). Like the oil in your car, it reduces the friction between moving parts. The entire joint is encased in a protective bag called the capsule and is prevented from stretching too far by ligaments—bands of fibrous tissue that bind two bones at the joint.

Other tissues such as tendons, bursae, blood vessels, nerves, and lymphatics make up the anatomy of a joint, too. Muscles are not a part of the joint, but are connected to it by tendons. The tension exerted on joints by muscles can greatly affect function. The "use it or lose it" principle applies to joints as well as to muscles. If you don't use your muscles, they can shrink and weaken. The same thing happens to joints. But with regular exercise, muscles and joints can stay strong.

> *Joints, like snow, stay free from damage when loads are spread more evenly.*

Uneven stress placed on your joints can do a lot of damage. Imagine that you and a friend are walking in deep, powdery snow. You're wearing cowboy boots. Every time you take a step, you sink thigh-deep in the snow. But your friend, who is wearing snowshoes, can walk over the snow without making so much as a dent. That's because the snowshoes increase the surface area over which your friend's weight is distributed. Joints, like snow, stay free from damage when loads are spread more evenly. Yet if the load is concentrated in a single spot, there's an uneven stress. This is the basic problem with joints—any change in structure can lead to abnormal load forces on cartilage, starting the process of degenerative joint disease.

Throughout your life, joints are continually being rebuilt in response to stresses placed on them. The construction material for this process comes from the nutrients in food. As you'll see later, proper nutrition is vital for the growth, repair, and healing that takes place in joints.

Bones
More Than Just a Framework

■ Bone is a complex, living tissue. The 206 bones in your body work together with muscles and connective tissue to support, anchor, and protect vital organs and other soft tissues. As part of the skeleton, bones give shape to your body and provide the levers for movement.

Bone is built in layers. This gives it strength and flexibility. Bones have the same "tensile strength" (ability to withstand being pulled part) as steel, yet are as flexible as fresh oak and have only one-third the weight of steel.

But bones are more than just scaffolding for the body. At the core of the bone, for example, is the blood-producing marrow encased in cylindrical sheets of bone tissue. It is here that red blood cells, white blood cells, and platelets are spawned.

Bone is well supplied with blood. Every time your heart beats, 10 percent of your blood is pumped to the bones. This provides bones with life-giving nutrients required for ongoing renewal and change.

Bone is also the storehouse for fat and minerals, particularly calcium. Day in and day out, calcium is deposited or withdrawn. This is the job of bone cells called osteocytes. In response to messages from hormones, osteocytes keep calcium levels in blood nearly constant. Proper calcium levels are vital for the healthy functioning of nerves and muscles.

When bone is damaged (fractured), osteocytes initiate a healing response in a matter of hours. After initial trauma is resolved, a soft callus (lump) is formed, uniting broken bone ends. The callus slowly hardens and decreases in size until healing is complete.

Bones have a direct relationship to joints' health. Bone directly underneath the cartilage in joints is called subchondral bone. This bone nourishes the cartilage with oxygen, water, and nutrients conveyed through microscopic channels. This supply route is vital for carrying building materials called "chondroprotective agents" from the bloodstream to the cartilage to the exact site where they are needed. Thanks to this intricate supply network, you can eat foods or swallow a pill containing nutrients, and the nutrients will go straight to your joints.

In osteoarthritis, there is a bony overgrowth (osteophytes) around joints. Osteophytes, rather than cartilage damage, might be the actual cause of osteoarthritic pain. Sometimes, the extra mass created by osteophytes can spread the stress on joints around, easing the force on cartilage. But since osteophyte formation is a change in joint structure, eventually it becomes detrimental to joint health.

Cartilage
Internal Shock Absorbers

■ Cartilage is plastic-like tissue found throughout the body. It is made up of thick bundles of fibrous protein (collagen). Like a tapestry, collagen fibers are woven vertically, horizontally, and diagonally to form the shape and size of cartilage. As cartilage begins to merge with bone, it becomes more calcified or hardened, forming a seamless bond with bone.

Unlike other body tissues, cartilage has no blood vessels, nerves, or lymphatics. This puts it at a disadvantage in receiving the basics of life: namely, oxygen, water, and nutrients.

Cartilage is a supporting structure in the body. You find it in the tip of your nose, the hard but flexible material of your ears, and as a component of spinal discs. The skeletal system of a developing fetus is cartilage. In infants and children, the growing parts of bones begin as cartilage and later become hardened into bone in a complex process called ossification.

Most cartilage is found in the joints, where it helps cushion joints every time you move, as part of the body's shock-absorbing system. (Subchondral bone and muscles are also shock absorbers.) Cartilage also provides a smooth surface for easy movement of the joints. Because of its unique molecular structure, cartilage is able to evenly distribute the mechanical loads on joints.

There are four major structural components of cartilage:

◆ collagen
◆ proteoglycans
◆ water
◆ cells (chondrocytes)

Understanding these will help you see how cartilage can be repaired from the ravages of osteoarthritis and other joint disorders.

Collagen
A Protein Girder

■ Collagen is the most abundant protein in the body, making up about 6 percent of your body weight. Found everywhere in the body, collagen is the major structural protein in humans. Each collagen fiber is constructed from three chains of amino acids twisted together like a rope over and over until large structures are made.

The collagen-making process depends on a steady flow of nutrients, including amino acids (protein), vitamin C, iron, copper, and manganese. If any of these are in short supply, the manufacture of collagen is impaired.

Another collagen component is sugar. The addition of specialized sugars to specific points on the collagen fiber determines its strength. If anything interferes with this deposit, then collagen strength is sapped. The cells won't even bother to make new collagen. As you'll see, certain nutrients can convert themselves into these essential sugars, and this enhances the repair of joints.

If you tried to tear apart a piece of collagen, you'd have a difficult time because of its enormous tensile strength. This gives cartilage the toughness and resiliency to spring back after being compressed.

Like a molecular girder, collagen gives shape to vital organs. It forms a fine scaffolding for organ cells and blood vessels so that they can arrange themselves into their characteristic shapes. Collagen literally holds us together.

Proteoglycans
Molecular Key to Cartilage Function

■ You've probably never heard of proteoglycans, yet they are an important although much overlooked molecule. Until recently, these molecules weren't studied much because the technology wasn't available. That has since changed, and now the very latest scientific knowledge on their structure and function reveals how important proteoglycans really are.

Proteoglycans have the consistency of half-set Jell-O. They fill up the extracellular spaces in cartilage not taken up by collagen. They sop up water and swell like a sponge. However, there's not enough space for the proteoglycans to hold all the water for which they are capable. This creates a natural swelling tension held in check by collagen. The swelling pressure is what gives cartilage its ability to absorb shock and resist compression.

Structurally, proteoglycans are a combination of protein and sugar. Specialized cells in cartilage (chondrocytes) obtain sugar from the subchondral blood vessels and manufacture special sugars. One is N-acetylglucosamine (NAG), and another is glucuronic acid. In a biochemical process, these sugars are linked together to make a molecule called hyaluronan (HI-yah-lure-AH-nan). Hyaluronan also gives the fluid in your joints its lubricating ability.

Hyaluronan molecules are much longer than typical molecules and form the backbone of proteoglycans. Dozens of proteoglycan subunits are attached to each hyaluronan molecule, forming a structure resembling ribs sticking out from a spine. The proteoglycan subunits fill up empty spaces between collagen girders in cartilage.

Each proteoglycan subunit contains a long, core protein to which are attached hundreds of long chains of specially modified sugars. These are called glycosaminoglycans (GAGs), the most important of which is chondroitin (kon-DROE-it-in) sulfate. The attachments of these GAGs to each core protein resembles bristles sticking out from a bottlebrush.

Cartilage is unique among other tissues because of its high content of GAGs. GAGs are manufactured *by* chondrocytes, including chondroitin sulfates, and are made *of* modified sugars. What makes GAGs unusual? It is their high sulfur content in the form of sulfates that give GAGs the ability to retain water, which is what makes cartilage so effective as a shock absorber. Indeed, the presence of sulfate in cartilage can be compared to the gel inserted within the soles of some types of running shoes for cushioning support.

Like collagen, GAG production in cartilage requires adequate amounts of certain nutrients. Those nutrients essential to the production of GAGs in cartilage are sugar, glutamine (an amino acid), sulfates (from sulfur amino acids), manganese, and vitamins A and C.

Another very important concept related to your joints is that for the repair of cartilage, GAG synthesis must take place before proteoglycan and collagen synthesis. Why? Cartilage rebuilding is only as good as its GAG synthesis. There is an intriguing possibility in all this: If GAG synthesis could be bolstered by nutrients, then it's conceivable that you can help joints repair themselves. Now you can understand and appreciate why GAGs, proteoglycans, and hyaluronan are so important for joint health. This will be explored more in Part Two.

Chondrocytes
The Cartilage Makers

■ The only cells present in cartilage are chondrocytes (KONN-dro-SITES). Their job is to produce and maintain cartilage. It's not an easy job, either. Remember, cartilage is a bloodless tissue, deficient in the oxygen and nutrients needed for growth.

Like bone, cartilage is remodeled throughout life. Chondrocytes send out enzymes to tear down collagen and proteoglycans, and replace them with new ones.

The remodeling process happens very slowly, however, because collagen is a tough protein to break down. Plus, chondrocyte metabolism is slow. It might take as long as four years to replace collagen and proteoglycans, or repair damaged cartilage, depending on the joint. Like tires going bald before you buy a new set, cartilage has plenty of time to be damaged by biochemical invaders called free radicals, as well as by mechanical stresses.

Even bone remodels faster than cartilage! This slow remodeling means joint healing and repair can also take a long time. Good news, however: A tiny percentage of collagen (5 percent) gets replaced every eight days. Indeed, there might yet be hope for faster repair of collagen in cartilage.

In osteoarthritis, chondrocytes turn into cellular Dr. Jekylls and Mr. Hydes. As Mr. Hydes, they overproduce the enzymes responsible for tearing down cartilage. As Dr. Jekylls, they simultaneously rebuild cartilage, although not fast enough. What makes chondrocytes so deranged? If we could answer that, we'd be on the road to finding a sure cure for osteoarthritis. Learning what makes chondrocytes shift into a rebuilding mode is the key. As you'll learn in Part Two, certain nutrients have the ability to shift chondrocytes into the repair mode, and tone down the enzymes that tear down cartilage.

Tendons and Ligaments
The Connectors

■ Tendons and ligaments are the body's connectors. They attach muscles to bones, bones to bones, or muscles to muscles. They're made of very thick connective tissues in which collagen fibers run parallel. This arrangement gives them the tensile strength needed to connect muscles and bones.

Tendons attach muscle to bones and are rope-like in structure. To get an idea of what a tendon is, run your hand down the back of your lower leg from your calf muscle to your ankle. Just above your ankle, you'll feel the Achilles tendon, a tough cord that connects the calf muscle to the heel.

Some tendons, called aponeuroses (AY-poe-nuyr-OWE-sees) are flat, since the muscles they connect are also flat. An example is the attachment of the large chest muscle to the breastbone.

Injuries involving tendons are usually at the point of attachment to the bone. Tendons can also be accidentally cut by sharp objects.

Ligaments connect bones to bones and are more flexible than tendons. The reason is that ligaments contain some elastin, a mesh-like protein. Like Spandex fabric, elastin can stretch, then snap back to its original shape. Elastin is also found in the skin, vocal cords, respiratory organs, large arteries, and spinal ligaments, among other places.

The cellular makeup of tendons and ligaments is similar. Both contain cells (fibroblasts), which are also found in other connective tissues (except bone and cartilage). Fibroblasts are very tough cells that can thrive outside the body in cell cultures. They play a role in healing and require an ample supply of nutrients.

Joint Capsules and Cavities

■ Your joints are covered with a tough capsule of thick connective tissue, made mostly of collagen. The capsule works like a girdle for the joint, holding everything in place—cartilage, ligaments, menisci, and bone. The cavity is a small open space that physically separates the cartilage on different bones in the joint.

The inside lining of the capsule is a tissue called the synovium (sigh-NO-vee-um). It has two layers. One contains nerves, lymphatics, and blood vessels, which supply the joint cavity and cartilage with nutrients.

The other layer has specialized cells called synoviocytes, ranging in thickness from one to four cells. These cells make synovial fluid (a joint lubricant containing hyaluronan), proteoglycans, and collagen, as well as important molecules called cytokines. Produced from dietary fat or proteins, cytokines let other cells communicate with each other. Cytokines play a role in accelerating or reversing arthritis, as we shall see later.

Synovial Fluid for Lubrication

■ Think of synovial fluid as crankcase oil for your body's moving parts. This remarkable lubricant is filled with nutrient-carrying proteins, glucose, oxygen, calcium, and other nutrients. Synovial fluid also contains a small amount of hyaluronan—just enough to give it a very slippery consistency so that your joints move around with very little friction.

Accessory Joint Tissues

■ Many other structures are associated with joints. These include menisci, bursae, tendon sheaths, and other tissues with special functions.

Like washers for the body, menisci are disk- or wedge-shaped pieces of connective tissue found in synovial joints such as the knee. Structurally, the meniscus is a mixture of cartilage and fibrous tissue. The meniscus can heal because it has a partial blood supply. Until recently, this tissue was thought to be useless and was removed when damaged. We now know that removal leads to premature arthritis.

Bursae are sac-like membranes filled with a type of synovial fluid. They act as a ball bearing for the body, making it easy for muscles, skin, and connective tissue to glide smoothly over joints. Repetitive activity and overuse can damage or inflame the bursae causing a condition known as bursitis.

Tough, fibrous material called tendon sheaths wrap around tendons that have large ranges of motion. Their job is to protect tendons from damage during movement. Special cells lining tendon sheaths secrete hyaluronan to help lubricate moving tendons.

Throughout the synovium and joint capsule are blood vessels, nerves, and lymphatic vessels. These carry vital materials such as nutrients and immune system cells to the joints. Loose connective tissue and fat are next to the joint as well. These tissues play a role in joint healing and inflammation.

Preserving Joint Health

■ Joints don't work well when they're overused or underused. Either scenario can take its toll on joint health—to the point of accelerating cartilage breakdown. Fortunately, this process is both preventable and reversible. To understand how, let's examine the risk factors for osteoarthritis, described in the next chapter.

3

Osteoarthritis: Are You at Risk?

A retiree walks upstairs, and his joints snap, crackle, and pop like a bowl of Rice Krispies. A ballet dancer pirouettes with grace, only to misstep and break her ankle. The impact of a car accident jams a teenager's knee into the dashboard. A delivery driver for a furniture store improperly lifts and moves sofas, chairs, and tables, day in and day out.

Despite their different situations, what do all these people have in common? They're each at risk for developing osteoarthritis at some point in their lives. Age-related events, trauma, accidents, and repetitive work activities are all examples of circumstances that can lead to osteoarthritis.

Osteoarthritis sneaks up on the body slowly and gradually takes over. At first, it's barely noticeable. Then it rears its ugly head, and the pain is unbearable. Ignoring the symptoms and thus failing to reverse it early on only makes matters worse. Get to know the risk factors involved. That way, you can take control and nip this potentially disabling condition in the bud.

The Older You Get

■ Aging doesn't actually *cause* osteoarthritis. It only sets the stage for it. As you get older, some natural erosion in cartilage takes place—for several reasons. With age, bone changes it shape, muscles weaken, and neuromuscular reflexes slow down. These all put more stress on cartilage, causing it to disintegrate. Joint surfaces that were once separated by healthy cartilage in youth are now bumping and grinding in old age.

> *Aging doesn't actually cause osteoarthritis. It only sets the stage for it.*

Heart disease is a factor, too. It causes a progressive loss of circulation. Fewer nutrients are available to feed cartilage cells and the subchondral bone underneath. Cartilage can't rebuild itself and eventually becomes even more vulnerable to stress. The bone only gets harder, putting extra force on cartilage.

Severe osteoarthritis affects different joints at different ages. If you're between the ages of twenty-five and thirty-five, it strikes the big toe; between thirty-five and forty-five, the spine and the wrist. After age forty-five, you're likely to get osteoarthritis in the fingers and hand. The knees are the next target, usually after age fifty. By sixty years old and afterward, you start feeling the pain in your hips.

Taking a Hit from Trauma

■ Maybe you've already been told by the doctor that your old football injury will come back to haunt you as osteoarthritis later in life. Arthritis experts agree that any old injury to joints—whether from a car wreck, an occupational hazard, sports, or other trauma—can reappear as osteoarthritis.

Such examples of trauma are direct hits to the cartilage; others are not so obvious. Take deep-sea sponge divers, for example. Decompression from diving causes lots of microscopic bubbles to form in cartilage. These bubbles can actually break up cartilage. Even deep-diving dinosaurs and diving turtles have all shown joint damage from effects of these tiny air bubbles.

Hidden Signs of Damage

■ Suppose you've never had a traumatic injury. And you're not a deep-sea diver. Yet you've been diagnosed with osteoarthritis.

Clues to the cause lead us to the concepts of "repetitive motion" and "impulse trauma":

REPETITIVE MOTION

Certain activities, repeated over and over, stress the joints and lead to the eventual destruction of cartilage. Repetitive motion is a fact of life in many occupations.

Does this mean your job causes osteoarthritis? Although the evidence isn't clear-cut, repetitive motions on the job have been linked to osteoarthritis. So has hard physical labor, which puts stress on joints, leading to wear and tear. Farmers, miners, dock workers, and others in heavy labor occupations get osteoarthritis more often than do people in sedentary jobs. People who do heavy lifting—such as bus drivers and foundry workers—are three times more likely to develop osteoarthritis than those in desk jobs. (See table 3.1)

Do you use your hands a lot at work? If so, you might be at risk for developing osteoarthritis in your hands. Weavers are known to have more osteoarthritis in their right hands than in their left, a direct result of the weaving process. Interestingly, studies show that osteoarthritis of the hands is more common in the dominant hand.

So if you're right-handed, chances are you'll get osteoarthritis in that hand first. These findings support the notion that previous injuries and joint overuse contribute to osteoarthritis.

IMPULSE TRAUMA

This is a sudden, rapid blow to the joint. Slipping on ice, tripping off a curb, jumping up and landing awkwardly from a short distance—these are examples of movements that put a rapid force on the joint. There's not enough time for the muscles to absorb the shock of the impact. The force instead goes to the joint. Cartilage and subchondral bone bear the brunt of the blow.

But wouldn't jumping out of a tree be more stressful to the joints than tripping off a curb? In reality, a longer fall gives the muscles more time to resist and absorb the force, as well as distribute it more evenly over the joints. Dangerously high falls, however, altogether overload the body's shock-absorbing capabilities.

Another form of impulse trauma has to do with "minor muscular incoordination"—something that happens in more than one-third of all people under the age of thirty years. Let's say you're a runner, and you have minor muscular incoordination. This means your muscle fibers don't slow down your legs fast enough to properly distribute the load of a heel strike. The force goes to your knee joint instead. Drs. Kenneth Brandt and Henry Mankin, a pair of well-known rheumatologists, call this incoordination "microklutziness." It appears to be a significant risk factor for osteoarthritis. Studies have shown that 100 percent of all people with pre-osteoarthritic knee pain have minor muscular incoordination.

Free Radicals and Joint Damage

■ Free radicals are tiny molecules or atoms with unpaired electrons. They are formed by a combination of the body's own metabolism as well as exposure to pollutants, bacteria, radiation, and cancer-causing chemicals. In a move that damages cell membranes, free radicals latch on to other molecules in order to find a mate. This sets up a chain reaction that creates many more free radicals.

When there's a skirmish by free radicals at cell membranes, cells can be damaged, even destroyed, leaving them vulnerable to disease. In fact, free radicals are believed to account for—or at least speed up—the aging process, cancer, heart disease, and many other life-threatening conditions.

The chain reaction set off by free radicals might be at the root of certain immune system disorders, including rheumatoid arthritis. In rheumatoid arthritis, free radicals are produced by the body's immune system, whose own cells, acting like misguided missiles, assault the cartilage in joints.

There's conclusive evidence of free radical mischief in people with both rheumatoid arthritis and osteoarthritis. Levels of "lipid peroxides" (remnants of the fatty molecules from free-radical damaged cell membranes) are higher in the blood of rheumatoid arthritis and osteoarthritis patients than in healthy people.

Inflammation sets off free-radical production by activating immune system cells. These cells then migrate to damaged joints and begin making more free radicals. Inflammation also causes synovial cells to produce free radicals.

Another possible cause of free-radical production in joints has to do with "ischemia" (a lack of oxygen in tissues). Every time cartilage is overloaded, it is squashed. Once the load is released, the cartilage springs back to its original shape, soaking up synovial fluid like a sponge. This happens every time you take a step, jog down a track, or throw a baseball. As cartilage is squashed, it's momentarily cut off from oxygen, causing ischemia. When oxygen-rich synovial fluid is sopped up, free radicals are produced.

It's possible that the same process can happen even while you're sitting still! If your joints are out of mechanical kilter, a small area of cartilage in joints gets compressed. Ischemia occurs, and free radicals are formed.

Regardless of where free radicals are made, they're very destructive to joint tissues. Many studies have even found that these mischievous molecules attack the hyaluronan in synovial fluid. This causes a breakdown in the fluid's lubricating properties. Free radicals can also chip off pieces of collagen and GAGs from cartilage itself.

Where joints are concerned, free radicals do most of their damage in rheumatoid arthritis. Yet damage at any level is enough to set off the downward spiral of cartilage degeneration. That being so, free radicals might be as much the bad guys in osteoarthritis as they are in rheumatoid arthritis. This will have important implications when we look at antioxidant nutrients.

What About Gender?

■ We know that women are more prone to osteoarthritis than men. Over the age of fifty-five, more women than men have osteoarthritis. The disease becomes more severe in women, with four times as many joints involved. Yet it isn't a "woman's disease." Actually, no age group is immune. Under age forty-five, more men have osteoarthritis than women do. Osteoarthritis tends to strike women more often in the fingers and knees; men, the big toe and hip joint.

Osteoarthritis Hits You Where You Live

■ The worldwide incidence of osteoarthritis varies widely. Among world populations, Greenland Eskimos have a relatively low rate of osteoarthritis. Interestingly, they eat a diet rich in fish oils, namely omega-3 fatty acids, which appear to have protective effects on joints. In those Eskimos who become "westernized," the rate of osteoarthritis triples.

Many people afflicted with osteoarthritis believe warmer climates make the symptoms more bearable. This might help explain the popularity of retirement havens such as Arizona and Florida. There's no proof, however, that warmer temperatures affect who gets osteoarthritis.

Is Exercise a Risk Factor?

■ For years medical authorities have suggested that exercise—an occupation for some and a lifestyle for others—might put so much wear and tear on the joints that osteoarthritis eventually results. With so many people running, pumping iron, and doing aerobics, you'd expect droves of exercisers in doctors' offices having their joints examined. But the good news is that exercise itself does not cause osteoarthritis and in fact might help protect against it.

Experts generally agree that injuries related to exercise and sports can contribute to osteoarthritis later in life. A good rule of thumb is that if working out or playing sports causes joint pain of any kind, don't do it.

Can Ill or Injured Joints Be Repaired?

■ Maybe you think you'll never be able to walk through your garden. Or stroll down the sidewalk. Or quilt a comforter for your granddaughter. Or again play the guitar.

Your doctor says it's hopeless (not your musical abilities, your joint problems).

But is it?

Some compelling evidence says not–that osteoarthritis is, instead, reversible. Let's look at some facts and dispel a few myths in the process:

FACT NO. 1

Osteoarthritis is not inevitable. Some people never get it. Autopsies on people ninety years or older have shown this to be true. Plus, 10 percent of the population is completely spared from joint degeneration. Something in their metabolic makeup allows cartilage to repair itself, although we can't yet pinpoint what. But this much is clear: Cartilage can be repaired.

FACT NO. 2

Spontaneous remissions do happen. Often called "miracles," spontaneous remissions–unexplained but complete cures–have been observed and reported among osteoarthritis patients. This is more proof that cartilage can repair itself.

FACT NO. 3

Taking the load off joints reverses osteoarthritis. Broken limbs, paralysis, strokes–these unfortunate, often tragic circumstances force patients to rest or not use parts of their bodies. A curious thing happens, however: Not using an arthritic limb halts the progression of osteoarthritis. Studies have proved this.

Is there a way to take the load off afflicted joints, short of not using them? Yes. A surgical technique called osteotomy rearranges bone in an alignment more favorable to reversing osteoarthritis. (See chapter 12.)

FACT NO. 4

Juvenile chronic arthritis can be stopped. Children with this disease get better with certain types of exercise, namely chronic passive motion. It slows, even prevents, the progression of juvenile chronic arthritis. Damaged cartilage is fixed, under the right conditions. If this form of arthritis can be stopped using special exercise, it follows that maybe osteoarthritis can be helped.

An Incurable Disorder—Or Is It?

■ Although there's no known drug that actually reverses osteoarthritis, there's a whole arsenal of natural weapons you can use against it. They're nutrients–and they work. Many are being used in other countries with promising results. Examples are chondroprotective agents, which include some familiar names such as vitamin C, and some not-so-familiar ones such as glucosamine.

All these nutrients can be easily obtained from food or from nutritional supplements. What you need is the information to use them wisely. Part Two and Part Three will give you that information. Not only that, you'll be able to apply this knowledge and use it with your physician to complement your current medical treatment.

Keep in mind that nothing is a cure-all. The body, however, has a built-in ability to heal its own joints. Specific nutrients can actually maximize the body's own healing response.

Most people think of nutrition as the food we eat. But there's more to it than that. Nutrition is about how our bodies digest food, absorb digested food, and use it for "metabolism." In metabolism, cells replace cells, tissues repair themselves, and vital organs adapt to meet biochemical requirements. In sum, metabolism is the process that turns food into fuel for activity and renewal.

Nutrients from the breakdown of food have the power to re-build cells, renew the body, repair damage, prevent disease, even reverse the course of disease. In fact, single nutrients are now known to have specific health-building benefits. These nutrients are called nutraceuticals (NEW-trah-SOO-tick-uhls). There's sufficient scientific evidence showing that nutraceuticals—single nutrients or mixtures of nutrients—can actually turn up the healing and repair power of your joints, whether they're injured or diseased. With proper nutrition on your side, your prognosis isn't gradual deterioration, it's gradual improvement.

Osteoarthritis in Different Occupations

(Each occupation was compared to a sedentary control group)

	Osteoarthritis Incidence (percent)	
Occupation	**Those in Occupation**	**Control Group**
Farmers (all sites)	33	19
Miners (shoulder)	52	12
(knees)	46	32
(hips)	43	28
Dock workers (fingers, elbows, knees)	21	9
Shipyard workers (knees)	3.9	1.5

TABLE 3.1

PART TWO

Reversing Arthritis with Nutrients

4

Glucosamines: The Key Breakthrough for Joint Health

Molly is a poster child for the Arthritis Foundation. She developed a severe case of juvenile rheumatoid arthritis when she was two and a half years old. Molly's joints became so sore and swollen that she had to be carried out of bed each morning. She lost her appetite and stopped growing. She started to bleed internally and needed transfusions. Meanwhile, Molly's doctors made heroic efforts to control the pain and inflammation. Those efforts included administration of almost every possible drug used for rheumatoid arthritis. For another two years, Molly was unable to play or run, or just generally have fun like other children. Even with the finest medical care, Molly still had severe, life-threatening flare-ups.

As it turned out, Molly's godfather was a veterinarian, familiar with chondroprotective agents. Some are extracts of cartilage that are licensed as drugs to treat joint problems in animals (but not people) in the United States. After a long search, he suggested that Molly start taking a product called Cosamin, which contains glucosamine and chondroitin sulfates.

When she was five years old, and with her doctor's consent, Molly started taking six capsules daily. Within one week, Molly was getting out of bed by herself, without pain. After three weeks, Molly was playing, running, and eating like other kids, at an age when she was predicted to be in a wheelchair.

As of four months later, Molly was taking two capsules of Cosamin daily and had had no flare-ups. She is growing again, and quite happy. Medical tests for inflammation, which had previously been highly elevated, were now in the normal range. Molly is working with her physician to decrease drug dosages so that side effects can be diminished.

While at the national Arthritis Foundation meeting, Molly met Christy, another child the same age with juvenile rheumatoid arthritis. Like Molly, Christy had frequent, life-threatening flare-ups, which were barely controlled with high doses of medications. Unfortunately, the high doses of drugs were beginning to have their own dangerous side effects. Christy's arthritis had different symptoms from Molly's. She had very high fevers, skin rashes, and heart damage, along with joint pain.

After meeting Molly and learning of Molly's prescription to pain-free progress, Christy started taking six capsules of Cosamin daily. Within a week, her joint pain was gone. After three weeks, she showed no evidence of joint damage after medical examination. Because of side effects, Christy's doctors were forced to discontinue all anti-arthritis medication. This time, she did not have the life-threatening flare-ups which had routinely occurred before when she reduced her drug dosages. As was the case with Molly, Christy's laboratory tests for inflammation showed a return to normal values. Now Christy runs, plays, and enjoys life.

Equally astounding is the story of Mr. B., who suffers from Prieurn-Griscelli Syndrome (PGS), a very rare and deadly form of arthritis. PGS usually cripples by age ten and is fatal by age twenty. Mr. B. is twenty-five years old and still walking. Along with extensive medical treatments, Mr. B. has been taking

Cosamin. He feels that Cosamin has kept him from being crippled, because he worsens whenever he stops taking it.

These are but a few of the remarkable stories being attributed to chondroprotective agents in real-life settings. Another is the story of Dr. Larry Bader, who wrote the foreword for this book. Although these stories sound dramatic, no one is claiming that joint diseases can be cured by special nutrients. However, it's becoming increasingly apparent that specific nutrients have helpful effects on joint health, and people's well-being. You will see scientific evidence of this later in this chapter.

Joint Regeneration and Glucosamine

■ These remarkable stories have one thing in common: they center around a chondroprotective nutraceutical called glucosamine (glue-KOSE-ah-mean). Although relatively new to medical science, glucosamine is very familiar to our joints and connective tissues. Glucosamine is an important component without which our bodies cannot live.

What makes glucosamine so special for joint health? That's easy. Glucosamine is a modified sugar molecule manufactured by cells in our body. Glucosamine is the single most important component and precursor for GAGs. In fact, hyaluronan is half glucosamine. Chondroitin sulfate is half galactosamine, which is made directly from glucosamine. Collagen production also requires glucosamine. Cartilage cells (chondrocytes) manufacture glucosamine from glucose (blood sugar), and from a common amino acid called glutamine.

If our joint cells can make glucosamine, then why do we need to take extra amounts? Can't our chondrocytes simply make more glucosamine when they need to repair cartilage? No. During joint degeneration and arthritis, chondrocytes have been "told" to destroy cartilage. Manufacture of new cartilage cannot keep pace with the destruction. In severe joint damage, chondrocytes have been told to stop making glucosamine. Why? Some of the culprits might be "bad" cytokines and prostaglandins, which act as biochemical traitors that lead to cartilage degradation.

The advantage of taking glucosamine as a dietary supplement is that it can be grabbed by chondrocytes and used to build more cartilage. Perhaps even more importantly, there is good evidence that extra glucosamine can flip a switch and convince chondrocytes to stop destroying cartilage, and even rebuild it.

Glucosamine can do this because it is almost completely absorbed from the gut into the bloodstream. Like other nutrients, some glucosamine finds its way to synovial fluid and subchondral blood vessels, where it diffuses into cartilage. There, chondrocytes eagerly take up glucosamine, so manufacture of new GAGs and collagen can begin.

Once inside the chondrocyte, the real fun begins. Glucosamine is what is known as a *rate limiting* step. This means that chondrocytes determine whether or not they can make more cartilage by how much glucosamine is around. More glucosamine, more cartilage repair. Less glucosamine, less cartilage repair.

In this way, the glucosamine you swallow in a pill can convince your chondrocytes to rebuild, repair, and maintain healthy joints. Picture chondrocytes like little biochemical factories. Their job is to produce GAGs and collagen, and assemble them into cartilage. Normally, enough glucosamine is available to fill orders, and cartilage can be maintained in good health without need for extra supplies. But stresses from injuries or arthritis mean that chondrocytes cannot produce enough glucosamine, and degeneration results. (Remember how chondrocytes have two strikes against their metabolism because there are no blood vessels in cartilage?) If a shipment of extra glucosamine in the form of oral supplementation comes in early enough, the factory can keep up with demand, and cartilage can be maintained.

To illustrate this key concept, when glucosamine was added to cartilage cultures, GAG production increased by 170 percent! No other nutrients, drugs, or chemicals have been able to boost factory output like glucosamine.

Glucosamine and Joint Repair: The Evidence

■ Now that we know how glucosamine works inside our joints, let's see how well it works in real life. The evidence supporting glucosamine is impressive, so it is worthwhile to examine it in detail. This way, both you and your doctor will be convinced that glucosamine is a major breakthrough for joint health.

Most of the medical research on glucosamine and osteoarthritis originated in Europe. Pharmaceutical companies there were quick to understand the importance of glucosamine and, subsequently, file for patent protection. This allowed them to conduct research sooner than American companies.

One of the first reports came from Drs. Crolle and D'este, from the First Medical Division in Venice, Italy. In 1980 they studied thirty elderly patients (more than seventy years old), hospitalized with advanced osteoarthritis. For three weeks, half were given both injections and pills of glucosamine sulfate, while the other half were given both injections and pills of a standard painkiller. Both treatments showed large decreases in joint pain and improvements in joint functions. However, after treatments were stopped, glucosamine-treated subjects continued to improve, while the control subjects did not. In fact, four subjects given glucosamine became symptom-free, but none of the control group did! This study showed that even in severe degenerative joint disease, glucosamine could reduce pain as well as potent painkilling drugs, even in the relatively short time span of three weeks.

Another trial was reported by Dr. Jose Pujalte and colleagues from the National Orthopedic Hospital in Manila, the Philippines. Twenty people, each about sixty years old, with established osteoarthritis of the knee were studied. Half were given fifteen hundred milligrams of glucosamine sulfate daily for eight weeks, while the other half (controls) were given an inert placebo (sugar pill). All received standard medical care. After eight weeks, the glucosamine-treated subjects had far superior reductions in joint pain, swelling, and tenderness, with improvements in restricted movements. The authors were so pleased with the results that they recommended glucosamine be used to treat all patients with osteoarthritis. This study also suggests that glucosamine can make current treatments work even better.

Perhaps the most significant study on glucosamine and osteoarthritis was performed by Dr. Drovanti and colleagues at Vigevano General Hospital in Pavia, Italy. Eighty patients, each about sixty years old, were put into the hospital for thirty days. They had osteoarthritis of the neck, lumbar spine, or multiple joints. These are the toughest kinds of osteoarthritis to deal with. All subjects received rest and physical therapies, but no drugs. Half of the subjects were given fifteen hundred milligrams daily of glucosamine sulfate, and the other half were given sugar pills as the control group. Again, as in the other studies, big improvements were found for the glucosamine-treated group. Ten became symptom-free. No such improvements were seen for the control subjects.

Can Glucosamine Reverse Arthritis?

■ This study is important for another reason: direct, physical evidence of the ability of oral glucosamine to regenerate damaged cartilage. Near the end of the study, samples of cartilage were taken from a few subjects after accidents or surgery. The cartilage samples were examined by scanning electron microscopy, a powerful tool for visualizing the appearance of cartilage. Damage and destruction of cartilage typical of osteoarthritis were found from two control subjects. However, cartilage from two glucosamine-treated subjects looked like it was from young, healthy people! Since all subjects had bad osteoarthritis before glucosamine, the most likely explanation for the results seen was that glucosamine actually reversed cartilage damage.

Indeed, the authors stated: "According to our scanning electron microscopy findings, glucosamine sulfate appears to rebuild the damaged cartilage. It would therefore appear to be the appropriate treatment to attack the underlying cause of the osteoarticular degenerative disorders." (*Clinical Therapeutics* [1980] Volume 3, pages 260-272).

This study is extremely important because there is practically no evidence in the medical literature that anything can *reverse* osteoarthritis. The results of all the studies on animals and people offer supporting evidence that glucosamine can rebuild damaged cartilage. Now we have direct evidence. This is the major breakthrough for joint health we have all been looking for.

Comparing Glucosamine to Drugs

■ Another study conducted in 1982 by Dr. Antonio Vaz, of St. John's Hospital in Oporto, Portugal, compared glucosamine sulfate to ibuprofen head-to-head. Forty subjects with knee osteoarthritis were given either fifteen hundred milligrams daily of glucosamine sulfate, or twelve hundred milligrams daily of ibuprofen for eight weeks. During the first two weeks, ibuprofen gave better relief from pain. After two weeks, ibuprofen did not help further. By eight weeks, glucosamine-treated subjects had *less* pain than the ibuprofen group and showed better improvements in joint functions. Thus, a direct comparison between the most commonly used drug for osteoarthritis and glucosamine was clearly in favor of the nutrient.

Doctors Rate Glucosamine

■ A more down-to-earth type of study was reported in 1982. Results of oral glucosamine sulfate treatment for an entire country, Portugal, were compared to other drug treatments for osteoarthritis. This means that glucosamine treatment for osteoarthritis was already an acknowledged standard treatment. Over a nine-month period, 252 doctors treated each of 1,506 osteoarthritis patients with fifteen hundred milligrams of glucosamine sulfate daily for six to eight weeks. Ninety-five percent of the people had good or sufficient overall results, as rated by their doctors. In comparison, 1,077 people treated with NSAIDs (like ibuprofen) or corticosteroids showed only a 70-percent success rate.

Thus, doctors rated oral glucosamine better for treating osteoarthritis than other standard drugs, cartilage extracts (covered in the next chapter), or vitamins. (I can see the advertisements coming up in the near future: "Nine out of ten doctors recommend glucosamine for their patients who have bad knees.") The authors concluded: "The results of this investigation . . . leads us to conclude that ambulatory oral treatment with glucosamine sulphate manages most arthrosis patients to full or partial recovery, whatever the localization of their arthrosis, concomitant illnesses or treatments . . ."

Finally, 1992 reports emanating from Rotta Research Laboratories in Monza, Italy, again found that glucosamine sulfate was superior to placebo, and just as good as ibuprofen for pain reduction and improvement of joint movements. In this series of studies, 606 subjects were studied in well-controlled trials.

It can be concluded that the consensus of medical research on clinical use of glucosamine for osteoarthritis is overwhelmingly positive. Every single study showed good results from taking oral glucosamine on joint health, *without side effects.* The available evidence also suggests that glucosamine can do something that no drug can: Glucosamine can actually *reverse* osteoarthritis! We have seen that glucosamine works by giving joints what they are hungry for—specific building blocks.

> *Every single study showed good results from taking oral glucosamine on joint health, without side effects.*

Does this mean that aspirin and NSAIDs are obsolete for treating osteoarthritis? Although it may be tempting to say yes, the rapid pain relief offered by these drugs is something that people want at any cost. Since these drugs are relatively inexpensive, it might be wise to use them at modest doses during the initial treatments for osteoarthritis. It seems that they work very well along with glucosamine, and no interactions are suspected. More information on NSAIDs will be presented later in this book.

Glucosamine and Sports Injuries

■ Mark, a black belt in Japanese martial arts, complained of a chronically sore elbow and wrists. Ibuprofen just wasn't working.

Although skeptical, he started taking six capsules of Cosamin a day. A tournament was coming up in three weeks and he wanted to participate.

By tournament time, he was pain-free (much to the chagrin of his opponents). In Mark's case, minor joint injuries seemed to be helped by taking Cosamin.

My wife Naniece is an avid Jazzerciser who uses weights on her arms and legs during the routines. Recently, her class moved to a new facility with considerably harder floors. After a few weeks, she had sore knees that got downright painful when she walked up and down stairs.

Naniece started taking six capsules of Cosamin daily. Within just three days, the pain was gone and she never skipped a class. After a week, she discontinued the supplement and was fine for about six months. Then the familiar knee pain returned. Naniece started Cosamin again. After a week, the pain disappeared. It hasn't returned since. Naniece's case demonstrates the power of a glucosamine product in enhancing healing of joint injuries in early stages. It made all the difference in her performance and joint health.

News from the medical front also supports the use of glucosamine for joint injuries. Dr. D. Böhmer and colleagues, from Frankfurt, Germany, looked at the effects of glucosamine sulfate supplements on sixty-eight young athletes with severe jumper's knee. The athletes took fifteen hundred milligrams of glucosamine sulfate for forty days, followed by seven hundred fifty milligrams a day for the next ninety to one hundred days. Four weeks after the athletes started using glucosamine, their knee pain was almost completely gone. By eight weeks, pain was completely gone. After four to five months, the athletes were training at their pre-injury intensities with no ill effects. Follow-ups one year later showed complete success with no problems.

Glucosamine and Wound Healing

■ Researchers from Columbia University in New York City discovered that glucosamine applied directly to surgical wounds of rats made the wounds heal 10 percent faster. Although this might not sound like much, there aren't too many substances that can speed surgical healing at all.

When chitin (the outer skeleton of crabs, lobsters, and insects) was applied to surgical wounds, they healed a remarkable 30 percent faster! It just so happens that chitin is a polymer made up of glucosamine. The researchers figured that chitin stayed put in healing tissues, making glucosamine readily available on an as-needed basis by enzymes normally associated with the healing process. This series of experiments mirror the results seen by adding glucosamine to cartilage cultures. In other words, if enough glucosamine is made available to healing tissues, recovery can be enhanced.

Glucosamine, Inflammation, and NSAIDs

■ Numerous studies in animals have proven that glucosamine is *not* a painkiller like aspirin or NSAIDs. So how can the results of clinical trials be explained, where glucosamine-treated people had less pain? It is now apparent, from animal studies, that glucosamine may be an anti-inflammatory nutrient. Glucosamine does not work the same way as aspirin, NSAIDs, or corticosteroids. Instead, at high doses, glucosamine inhibited free-radical production and decreased the amount of damaging enzymes released during inflammation. Although it is not yet known exactly how glucosamine does this, it might be due to the ability of glucosamine to convince cells to repair rather than destroy.

The net result would be less inflammation, which is what the studies showed.

This concept was verified when oral glucosamine given to rats prevented arthritis produced by chemicals. These models of arthritis mimic rheumatoid arthritis in humans, which might explain the remarkable results of Molly and Christy (and others) with juvenile rheumatoid arthritis. Unfortunately, there are no controlled clinical studies of glucosamine effects on rheumatoid arthritis.

As we will see later, the most commonly used drugs to relieve pain in arthritis might actually *inhibit* cartilage repair. Perhaps glucosamine can come to the rescue. Studies using cartilage cultures showed that glucosamine sulfate could partially reverse the damage caused by aspirin and NSAIDs (including ibuprofen). This is a very important concept, since millions of people are using rather high doses of aspirin and NSAIDs for long time periods. Also, combining glucosamine with painkilling drugs might accentuate the benefits of each and reduce side effects associated with drugs. This situation definitely needs more exploration.

Too Good to Be True?

■ All this research and information makes glucosamine look fantastic for joint health. In fact, glucosamine is the first-line drug of choice for treating osteoarthritis in several European countries. The research is solid and convincing. Although one can always say more research is needed before glucosamine can be recommended here in the United States, the same can be said of almost every drug. The bottom line is that plenty of good research on humans has been performed over many years, and the research overwhelmingly points to the safety and effectiveness of oral glucosamine. If this is true, then why have we not heard about this wonder nutrient? Is glucosamine too good to be true?

At this time, the FDA does not accept foreign studies for approval of a new drug in the United States. Also, since glucosamine is already a nutrient, it is very difficult from a legal perspective to file an application to make glucosamine into a drug. Because glucosamine products are already available as food supplements, and the new drug approval process is costly and time-consuming, no company in their right economic mind would dare attempt turning glucosamine into a drug. You probably won't see glucosamine as an approved drug in this country for many years. This does not mean that glucosamine does not work or is illegal.

Does this mean you can't get or use glucosamine? Quite the contrary. Doctors have the right and privilege to use whatever they see fit to treat patients. Thus, your doctor can recommend that you take glucosamine. If you are sufficiently educated, you might purchase glucosamine as food supplements for whatever purpose you wish. As long as manufacturers do not make drug claims for their nutrient products, glucosamine is perfectly legal for sale.

Of course, it is rather difficult to talk about glucosamine without making drug-like claims. This reflects the outdated nature of our Food, Drug, and Cosmetic Act. Back in the thirties, it was generally believed that foods were foods and could not affect health or diseases. Therefore, drugs were set up to fix diseases. Anything that could affect the body was legally classified as a drug to better protect consumers from rampant quackery, which was prevalent at the time. However, the concept that food does not affect health is dead wrong. So much evidence has piled up to support the use of foods and specific nutrients to assist health (in essence, be drugs), that the laws are now badly in need of revision. Fortunately, there are signs that the legal status of foods with medical uses is becoming more appropriate.

Glucosamine in Foods

▪ This brings us to the question of where to find glucosamine. Is there a food rich in glucosamine? How do I get enough glucosamine to do my joints any good?

Although almost all foods contain glucosamine, it is bound up in polymers such as proteoglycans, GAGs, collagens, and other proteins. No food is particularly rich in glucosamine, except maybe cartilage itself, which is not a very common dietary item. After all, how many of you have said: "Honey, I'm going to the store to get some raw beef trachea powder?" Not too many, I presume.

Also, glucosamine is probably mostly destroyed by cooking and heating. Even though nobody has analyzed foods for glucosamine content, it is very likely that regular dietary intake from foods is rather low. Getting glucosamine from foods in the diet is not practical.

Forms of Glucosamine Supplements

▪ The best way of getting glucosamine is through dietary supplementation. This brings us to the question: What's the best glucosamine supplement to take?

Three kinds of glucosamine are commercially available:

◆ glucosamine hydrochloride
◆ glucosamine sulfate
◆ N-acetylglucosamine (NAG)

To make a long story short, what you want is glucosamine. It does not matter if glucosamine has sulfate, hydrochloride, or Kalamazoo attached to it. There is no practical difference between any of the forms of glucosamine in supplement products.

This was proven in cartilage culture studies. They will all work equally well, as long as the same amount of glucosamine is given. This is where differences start.

When pure, glucosamine slowly breaks down upon exposure to air and water. Pharmaceutical preparations used glucosamine hydrochloride to stabilize glucosamine sulfate. However, an independent analysis of glucosamine sulfate raw material available in America has shown that salt (sodium chloride) has been used as the stabilizer. Thirty percent of glucosamine sulfate supplements is salt.

Because sulfate accounts for 20 percent of the weight of glucosamine sulfate, this means that a typical supplement product labeled as five hundred milligrams of glucosamine sulfate per capsule might only contain two hundred fifty milligrams. You would have to take six capsules of the glucosamine sulfate supplement products to reach the amount used in clinical studies, not three capsules as the label would have you believe. You would also get nine hundred milligrams of sodium daily, which is not good news to people on salt-restricted diets.

Fortunately, glucosamine hydrochloride and NAG are available pure—without salt. However, NAG is metabolized differently from other forms of glucosamine. Within an hour after you take NAG, your liver and other tissues selectively grab it to make proteins. Less is available to cartilage.

This leaves glucosamine hydrochloride as the preferred form of glucosamine. It has a slightly higher concentration of glucosamine (83 percent, instead of 81 or 79 percent), better stability, better chance for an unambiguous label claim, and it's sodium-free.

But all the studies examined in this book used glucosamine sulfate. Is glucosamine hydrochloride going to work as well? The answer is yes, if not better. Animal and cartilage culture studies all showed that glucosamine hydrochloride was equal to or better than other forms of glucosamine in helping cartilage cells.

Some manufacturers claim that the sulfate part of glucosamine sulfate makes it the best choice. Don't believe them, because the sulfate is removed from the glucosamine during digestion and transport. The sulfate is excreted, and will not materially affect cartilage. Cartilage gets most of its sulfate for GAG synthesis from certain amino acids.

There is, therefore, no advantage to blending several kinds of glucosamine salts in one product. You might find supplement products that combine glucosamine with other nutrients. This is commonly done by manufacturers to have a unique product so shoppers cannot easily compare prices. Unless there is a very good rationale for adding other ingredients to glucosamine, the net result is a more diluted glucosamine product.

There is one exception, however. It's Cosamin, a patented product described in the case studies in this chapter. Cosamin is a formulation with two hundred fifty milligrams of glucosamine hydrochloride, two hundred fifty milligrams of chondroitin sulfates (covered in the next chapter), and five milligrams of manganese (a mineral with important roles for joint health to be covered in another chapter) per capsule. The glucosamine hydrochloride is pharmaceutical grade, not available to the supplement market. Taking six capsules daily equals the amount of glucosamine used in the successful European trials discussed earlier.

You can obtain Cosamin from pharmacies or physicians. One pharmacy that sells Cosamin to individuals is Ritchie Pharmacy in Baltimore, Maryland (1-800-450-3620). Dr. Robert Kantorski, a doctor of pharmacy, is familiar with the product and can answer additional questions you might have.

Using Glucosamine Products

■ It's best to take glucosamine in the morning and evening (two divided doses a day). You can take it either with meals or on an empty stomach. Of course, it is preferred to use glucosamine under the guidance of your physician. Glucosamine products should not replace a physician's advice or other medical treatments. If you suspect a serious joint problem, please see your doctor. Glucosamine products and other nutritional therapies work in concert with standard treatments, and not alone unless recommended by your doctor. Remember that you are a partner with your doctor in determining the best course of treatments.

At first, take fifteen hundred milligrams of glucosamine daily until your symptoms have decreased. Then reduce your dosage to one thousand milligrams daily for two weeks. As your symptoms continue to improve, reduce the dosage to five hundred milligrams a day. Your goal is to manage your symptoms with the lowest amount of glucosamine necessary. If your symptoms disappear, you can stop taking it altogether. If symptoms return, simply increase dosage. Remember that glucosamine, being a foodstuff, has a flexible dosage schedule.

The cost for a one-month supply of glucosamine can range from thirty to sixty dollars, or about one or two dollars a day. That cost will fluctuate as dosages are decreased or increased. Thus, the cost of supplementing with glucosamine is comparable to taking some NSAIDs.

What to Expect

■ When can you expect to see results? This is a tough question to answer because everyone is different. Different body weights and the severity of your condition make predicting individual responses difficult. Ideally, you should note some improvements by two weeks and definitely by eight weeks. If there is no change or your condition worsens after eight weeks, chances are that glucosamine won't work well at that dosage level. At that point, you have two options: stop taking glucosamine or increase your dosage.

Glucosamine Safety

■ Is glucosamine safe? The answer is a resounding yes! Here is the evidence:

◆ No adverse side effects have been reported in the numerous patient-hours of human studies, including those mentioned in this chapter.

◆ In animal studies by Setnikar, glucosamine was found to be at least one thousand to four thousand times safer than indomethacin, a common NSAID prescribed for osteoarthritis.

◆ Other animal studies by Setnikar found no toxicity, even after feeding the human equivalent of one-third of a pound of glucosamine every day for over a year. This would be like taking several full bottles of glucosamine pills every day.

If you are pregnant or hope to become pregnant soon, consult your physician before using glucosamine. The effects of glucosamine supplementation on a growing fetus are not known. It's not worth taking even a tiny chance that something might happen.

In short, oral glucosamine appears to be extremely safe.

5

On the Mend with Chondroprotective Agents

If there was such a thing as a natural supplement that stops the breakdown of cartilage and stimulates its repair, wouldn't you want to take it for osteoarthritis? Wish granted. There is such a supplement, and it's called chondroitin (konn-DROE-it-in) sulfate. Chondroitin sulfates are the major GAG in cartilage and other connective tissues. As supplements, they're made from cow cartilage, shark cartilage, or whale cartilage. Some of the supplement's clinical reports sound truly amazing:

- ◆ In test tubes, chondroitin sulfates stimulated the production of cartilage–and arrested degradative enzymes that destroy it.
- ◆ In a German study, thirty-five patients with osteoarthritis took oral chondroitin sulfates for three months. In every person, joint mobility improved and pain was reduced.
- ◆ In several Italian studies, osteoarthritis sufferers reported less pain, less reliance on pain medication, and improvements in joint movement.

A Wonder Supplement?

■ This bright spot on the horizon of natural treatments for arthritis owes a debt to a group of chondroprotective drugs used in Europe since the sixties: Arteparon™, Rumalon™, and hyaluronan. All are purified or semi-purified components of cartilage. They're not taken orally, but instead are injected. In the United States, none are approved for use in humans, although some are approved for animals.

Arteparon and Rumalon were originally developed by Swiss and German pharmaceutical companies as heart drugs. As such, they were supposed to dissolve plaque in heart disease and thin the blood to prevent clot formation. Neither drug was too successful against heart disease. However, a funny thing happened: Doctors noticed that people with arthritis got better. Eventually, both drugs were approved for the treatment of arthritis in German-speaking countries. Millions of doses of these drugs have been given over the years. Let's look at them in more detail:

Rumalon has the longest history of clinical use. A true proteoglycan, it's formulated from an extract of cow cartilage and cow bone marrow. Rumalon is usually given as twenty injections into the muscle over a three-month period and repeated as needed.

Dozens of animal studies show that Rumalon prevents, stops, or slows the progression of arthritis. Other animal and test-tube studies demonstrate that Rumalon repairs cartilage and inhibits an enzyme called elastase, which chews up cartilage. Not only that, Rumalon reverses cartilage damage done by steroid and nonsteroid drugs.

Rumalon might produce some allergic reactions, however. Concern over this has limited its widespread use.

Arteparon is chondriotin sulfates extracted from cow cartilage, to which extra sulfates are synthetically attached. Numerous animal studies have shown that Arteparon slows down and stops cartilage destruction, thus preventing arthritis.

Like Rumalon, Arteparon is given to patients as a set of twenty intramuscular injections over a three-month period. Also like Rumalon, there is a concern over allergies. In fact, three fatalities in Europe from severe allergic reactions had been recorded as of late 1994. The drug has some anticoagulant effects, too, meaning that it thins the blood, occasionally too much. As a result of these side effects, interest in Arteparon has diminished in recent years.

Renamed as Adequan, the drug is approved in the United States for veterinary use to treat joint problems in horses. Some vets use it to treat small animals such as dogs, although the drug is not government approved for this use, except in Canada.

The Athletes' Edge?

■ If these drugs can put cartilage on the mend, shouldn't they also do the same for cartilage damage in athletes?

Several European studies have looked into this. In studies involving 2,002 athletes, Arteparon was used to treat cartilage damage in chronic joint injuries, including jumper's knee and tendinitis. Overall, between one-half and two-thirds of the athletes responded well, and many surgeries were prevented.

When the researchers compared Arteparon to conventional drugs, they found that it fared as well or better. Pain was reduced,

joint mobility improved, muscles got stronger, and athletes returned to activity faster—all after treatment with Arteparon. And
so the evidence hints at cartilage extracts being a beneficial treatment for sports injuries.

A Role in Osteoarthritis

■ Among the many studies that have been done on these drugs,
two stand out, both done by Dr. V. Rejholec of Prague,
Czechoslovakia, beginning in the mid-sixties. Dr. Rejholec knew
that cartilage can repair, but only very slowly. That being so, he
believed that any studies on chondroprotective agents and osteoarthritis should go on for many years to show proof of cartilage
repair. So that's what he did—and what no other study, even on
approved drugs, has done since.

At the time Dr. Rejholec conducted his studies, he lived in a
communist state. Everybody "enjoyed" socialized medicine.
Disability from osteoarthritis was such a costly problem that communist leaders were willing to give every consideration to cutting
health-care costs. Research into chondroprotective agents fit the
bill, in light of its potential to prevent expensive surgeries and get
people back to work.

In the first study, 112 patients with osteoarthritis of the hip
were given NSAIDs and physical therapy as standard treatment.
Half the group received fifty shots of Rumalon each year, while
the other half got fifty shots of vitamin B_{12} each year. Vitamin B_{12}
doesn't affect osteoarthritis and was used as a placebo.

Dr. Rejholec followed these patients for ten years. The data
was clearly in favor of the Rumalon group. Those patients took
half the NSAIDs that the controls took. X-rays of the hips revealed
that taking Rumalon slowed down the progression of joint damage. In fact, the number of patients with severe disease actually

decreased in the Rumalon group (from sixty to fifty-two), whereas joint damage increased among controls (sixty to sixty-eight). Seventeen controls needed hip-replacement surgery, compared to only six in the Rumalon group.

One of the most significant outcomes was the reduction in lost working days. Prior to the study, the patients were off work about forty working days a year. At the end of the ten-year study, the Rumalon-treated patients were able to return to work more often, losing between twenty and forty days out of each year. By contrast, the controls were out of work nearly one hundred eighty days every year. Rumalon treatment saved millions of dollars in health-care costs.

Dr. Rejholec's second study looked at the effects of Rumalon and Arteparon on osteoarthritis of the knee. In this five-year study, one hundred fifty patients underwent standard treatments, including NSAIDs and physical therapy. Fifty patients were treated with Arteparon, and fifty patients with Rumalon; the control group of fifty with placebos. Initially, everyone in the study felt less knee pain. But later, the controls started hurting again. After five years, they were in as much pain as when the study began. Those treated with Rumalon or Arteparon, however, had an entirely opposite reaction. By the end of five years, their pain was almost gone. They were able to cut down on their NSAIDs as well.

Other impressive findings followed. The Rumalon and Arteparon groups could walk up and down stairs with greater ease; the controls could not. Only two patients from the Rumalon and Arteparon groups had to have knee surgery, compared to thirteen controls.

At the start of the study, about three out of four patients from each group were too disabled to work. By the end of the study, all controls were off work. But half the people treated with

Arteparon were working after five years, and 80 percent of the Rumalon-treated group had returned to work.

Both studies offer clear proof that injectable chondroprotective agents have a profound effect on people with osteoarthritis. These effects didn't happen overnight, however. Fixing cartilage takes a long time. If the studies had lasted a month or two, it's unlikely any significant changes would have been observed. In fact, it's almost impossible to find studies on NSAIDs and osteoarthritis lasting longer than a few months. These studies underscore what researchers have known all along: NSAIDs don't stop the progression of osteoarthritis; instead, they might aggravate it.

The enlightening results of these studies have been largely ignored in the United States. In fact, they weren't even published in English until 1987. A lot of credit should be given to Dr. Rejholec, who devoted twenty years of his life to this work. He showed that simple extracts of cartilage, which were mostly chondroitin sulfates, could reverse the course of osteoarthritis.

Hyaluronan

■ Imagine how much easier life would be if you could get a lube job for creaky joints the same way you can for your car. That possibility isn't so far-fetched. Research on injecting hyaluronan into joints is going on now. As described in chapter 2, hyaluronan is the substance that gives synovial fluid its lubricating properties. You don't need to use a dipstick to know that arthritic joints are low on hyaluronan.

In a purified form, hyaluronan is approved for use in eye surgery for humans. As such, it replaces vitreous humor, which is a solution of hyaluronan found inside eyeballs. Successful research with animals led to the approval of hyaluronan for use by vets to treat animals with joint disease.

In human studies, hyaluronan injected into knee joints has shown promise by reducing pain and increasing range of motion. Hyaluronan has also been found to relieve symptoms of TMJ (a disorder of the jaw) better than do corticosteroid injections. In a Finnish study, researchers applied hyaluronan to torn or perforated eardrums. Remarkably, it repaired eardrums that had not healed for ten years. In most patients, hyaluronan sped up the healing of this delicate hearing organ.

Hyaluronan might also be able to prevent adhesions formed during the healing of severed tendons. Hyaluronan injected into rabbit knees enhanced the healing of torn ligaments. If the same could be done in humans, football players and other athletes could lead more pain-free lives.

The medical world is still mulling over the use of hyaluronan as a treatment for joint and connective tissue injuries. It's clear that hyaluronan has therapeutic value; however, a drawback is that it has to be injected. This may keep it from becoming popular as a chondroprotective agent.

> *In human studies, hyaluronan injected into knee joints has shown promise by reducing pain and increasing range of motion.*

Chondroprotective Nutrients

■ With chondroprotective drugs, it takes years to see results. Also, there's the potential for allergic reactions, and you have to get injections in or near the affected joint. Is there a way to get the therapeutic benefits of these drugs without the hassle? Yes—with chondroitin sulfates, a nutrient that's a close cousin to Rumalon, Arteparon, and Hyaluronan. Chondroitin sulfates are available as an oral supplement and have some proven benefits of their own.

Chondroitin sulfates were discovered almost by accident. When researchers sprinkled cartilage powder on healing bones and skin wounds, they found that wounds started healing better. Subsequently, a search ensued for the active healing ingredient in the cartilage powder. It turned out to be chondroitin sulfates. Further research into the nutrient's powers became a top priority.

One study examined a certain strain of mice that spontaneously gets osteoarthritis. Chondroitin sulfates were fed to the animals before they became arthritic. The result? Fewer arthritic joints–and a reduction of severe arthritis by about 25 percent. When conventional drugs were given to the mice, osteoarthritis got worse. Clearly, chondroitin sulfates had a protective effect.

What about studies in humans? Several have been conducted. Dr. John Prudden at Columbia University used injectable chondroitin sulfates (called Catrix-S) with twenty-eight osteoarthritis patients and found "excellent" results. Likewise, Dr. E. M. Kerzberg, from the department of medicine at J. M. Ramos Mejia Hospital in Buenos Aires, Argentina, observed that injecting chondroitin sulfates for twenty weeks into patients with osteoarthritis of the knee reduced pain and improved movement. Accumulating research continues to show that osteoarthritis sufferers respond to treatment with chondroitin sulfates.

Taking Chondroitin Sulfates to Heart

■ And so do heart patients. For forty years, Dr. Lester Morrison of the Loma Linda School of Medicine in Los Angeles studied the effects of chondroitin sulfates on heart disease. In a six-year study, one hundred twenty patients with atherosclerosis (hardening of the arteries) underwent standard treatment, but with one exception. Half the group took fifteen hundred milligrams of chondroitin sulfates daily for six years.

After six years, thirteen controls had died, compared to only four deaths in the chondroitin sulfate group. Also, in the control group, there were forty-two cardiovascular incidents, including heart attacks, strokes, and hospitalization—but only six in the chondroitin sulfates group. Somehow, chondroitin sulfates enhanced coronary health.

Despite the promising results, the FDA ruled that chondroitin sulfate was not a pure substance and could not be classified as a drug. Suppressing such good results on a trivial point seems hasty, especially in light of how chondroitin sulfates could potentially help the millions who suffer from heart disease, the number-one killer in the United States.

I bring up Dr. Morrison's work for two reasons. First, he proved that large, oral doses of chondroitin sulfates are well tolerated for long periods. Second, his work confirmed that chondroitin sulfates are absorbed through the small intestine and into the bloodstream, which eventually carries the nutrient to cartilage. Thus, chondroitin sulfates have the potential to be chondroprotective agents when taken orally. They don't have to be injected to produce improvement in joints. Furthermore, if you're taking chondroitin sulfates, your arteries might get healthier.

In fact, a product containing purified chondroitin sulfates and similar compounds is being tested in Europe to counteract senile dementia caused by hardening of the arteries. The product is called Ateroid, and so far, it has improved the mental function in almost nine thousand patients. The lessons taught by Dr. Morrison have not been lost at all; they've just moved to Europe.

A Personal Case Study

■ So intrigued by the evidence in support of chondroitin sulfates, I decided to test these nutrients on Koko, my five-year-old

Boston Terrier, which was afflicted with arthritis in her knee. She began walking with a limp, and before long, was holding up her leg. In short, we had a three-legged dog. Koko was faced with knee surgery. Instead, we opted to give her a daily dose of three hundred milligrams of chondroitin sulfates. We simply wrapped the capsule in a piece of American cheese, which she would never refuse. We had been giving her garlic oil capsules in the same manner, so a potential placebo effect was ruled out immediately.

After two weeks, Koko put her leg to the ground, but without much weight on it. In another two weeks, she put more weight on the leg. Then, two weeks later, she resumed her favorite pastime of chasing neighborhood cats. Muscle strength in her leg returned, and within a few months, she competed in a canine fun run without any discomfort. Koko's recovery astounded her vet, who had never seen such a remarkable transformation without surgery.

Using Chondroitin Sulfates

■ If you're interested in trying chondroitin sulfates, how much should you take? Based on human studies, a daily dose of one thousand milligrams (one gram) is effective. Because the nutrient stays in the bloodstream for about twelve hours, it's a good idea to split the dose in two—one in the morning and one at night.

The advantages of using oral chondroitin sulfates over injectable drug forms are clear: With oral doses, you can continually saturate your cartilage with chondroprotective nutrients. Injectables can only be given once in a while and don't stay in the joint tissue as long. The longer the nutrients are in the joints, the faster the results. Taking chondroprotective nutrients is safer and more convenient than having them injected. After experiencing results from oral chondroitin sulfates, you can reduce your dosage.

One final point about chondroitin sulfates: It's difficult to find a pure product. According to an independent analysis, purity can range from zero to 98 percent. Only one product I know of was rated as 98 percent pure, and that product is Cosamin, discussed in the previous chapter. Other chondroitin sulfate products are available in health-food stores, but there's no way of determining their purity, short of chemical analysis. You might want to try the supplement for a month, then see if you notice any benefits. If you do, then the product is potent.

6

Antioxidants against Arthritis

Let's start right off with, as you can see by the above title's alliteration, several case studies verifying why studying this chapter could help give you an "A" on your health-care report card:

◆ After taking four grams of vitamin C daily for several months, Dr. J. Greenwood reported that he had "cured his lower-back pain." He started recommending that his patients with degenerative-joint disease take daily oral doses of one to four grams of vitamin C. Most patients got relief from their symptoms.

◆ An avid mountain climber is told that the only hope for his lingering knee pain is to give up the sport. For nine months, he takes sixty-eight milligrams of vitamin E and one thousand micrograms of selenium every day. He's soon able to resume his favorite pastime—pain-free.

◆ A patient with severe bursitis of the knee suffers from pain, tenderness, and swelling. He's barely able to move his knee. Doctors suggest taking vitamin C containing bioflavonoids every four hours. Twenty-four hours later, the pain and swelling are much better; seventy-two hours later, the patient's knee is practically as good as new.

◆ Osteoarthritis sufferers in a German study were given either four hundred IUs (International Units) of vitamin E or a placebo. In six weeks, the vitamin-E-supplemented group felt less joint pain and had much greater joint mobility than the placebo group. Plus, the patients taking vitamin E relied less on painkillers.

Antioxidants to the Rescue

■ The common denominator in all these cases is a class of nutrients known as antioxidants. The big three for joints are:

◆ vitamin C (ascorbic acid)
◆ vitamin E (tocopherols)
◆ the trace mineral selenium

Other antioxidants used by the body include beta carotene, glutathione, glutathione peroxidase, superoxide dismutase, catalase, coenzyme Q10, cysteine, methionine, and numerous plant-deprived compounds.

Antioxidants are nutrients in the news. Almost every day, results of another study about antioxidants are reported by the mass media. Most offer evidence that antioxidants are health-promoting nutrients which we do not get enough of in our diets. Enough antioxidants are believed to lessen our chances of getting the major killer diseases such as cancer, heart disease, diabetes, and arthritis. There is even growing evidence to suggest that antioxidants might slow the aging process.

Antioxidants protect our cells from the oxidation that normally occurs as our bodies burn oxygen to live. A product of oxidation is free radicals, or very reactive pieces of molecules or atoms. Free radicals are normally produced by our bodies in certain metabolic reactions, inflammation, and by our immune system to kill invading microbes or cancerous cells. Free radicals are also produced during ischemia, which is the term used to describe a relative lack of oxygen in our tissues.

Free radicals are also found in our environment. Smoke (especially cigarette smoke), air pollution, water pollution, certain radiations, some drugs, some pesticides, and many other compounds all cause free radicals to be generated.

Free radicals are particularly nasty because they set off a chain reaction of damaging molecular events. Thus, one free radical spawns a whole slew of other free radicals, each leaving a damaged molecule in its wake.

This chain of events is much like tossing a hot potato from one person to another. With each toss, someone's hand is burned until the potato is caught by a person wearing insulated mitts. That person holds the potato until it cools off, ending the chain reaction of burned hands. Like the mitts, antioxidants neutralize free radicals.

Free radicals, and the process of oxidation, can corrode cells and their components, in much the same way as rust forms on metal (another type of oxidation). Cell membranes, proteins, DNA, and even cartilage structures themselves can be attacked and physically damaged by free radicals. Damage is prevented when antioxidants are available to sop up free radicals before they crash into too many friendly molecules.

But can antioxidants stop the ravage of free radicals in joint disease? It's a question that hasn't been fully answered. Most of the clinical research on people has been done in Europe, while most of the research in the United States has been conducted in test tubes and under the microscope. However, there's some very provocative data suggesting that antioxidants are helpful in treating osteoarthritis and other joint injuries. What's not yet clear though is how to use them and what to expect from treatment.

For now, let's take a look at some of the known data on antioxidants and degenerative joint disease.

A Case for Vitamin C

■ The most well known of all vitamins, vitamin C is usually associated with preventing colds. Your body can't make vitamin C, so you have to get it from your diet. Vitamin C is vital for the growth and development of connective tissue, particularly collagen. Without vitamin C, defective collagen is produced, and you can get a disease called scurvy. Its symptoms include bleeding gums, fragile skin, easy bleeding and bruising, poor wound healing, and loss of bones and teeth. British sailors used to get scurvy until it was discovered that eating citrus fruits could prevent it. Lime juice was then put on all British sailing ships, and British sailors became known as "limeys." Today, scurvy is practically unheard of in the United States.

In test tubes, vitamin C triggers the manufacture of collagen and proteoglycans by cartilage cells (chondrocytes). The amount of vitamin necessary for this is the equivalent of megadosing. This brings up some important questions about megadoses: How much vitamin C is actually retained by the body? How much is excreted?

The RDA, or recommended daily level of dietary vitamin needed to prevent scurvy, is sixty milligrams. At one hundred milligrams a day, the blood and cells quickly become saturated with vitamin C. As higher doses are taken, the kidneys dump the overflow into the urine. Sounds like megadoses are a waste, right? Don't be so sure.

The spaces between cells and tissues, outside the bloodstream, soak up a lot of vitamin C. These are the spaces that feed cartilage. Theoretically, it might be possible to supercharge cartilage and its cells with vitamin C, enhancing the synthesis of cartilage. This would be ideal for reversing degenerative joint disease.

Some interesting work with vitamin C and joint problems has emerged from one animal study done in 1984. At Tufts University in Boston, vitamin C was given to guinea pigs at doses of sixty times the guinea pig RDA before and after knee surgery. This dosage almost completely prevented osteoarthritis. The findings led researcher Dr. Edith Schwartz to state: "Judicious use of these vitamins in the treatment of osteoarthritis, either alone or in combination with other therapeutic means, may thus be of great benefit to the patient population by retarding erosion of cartilage."

In human terms, the experimental dose equals 3,750 milligrams a day. Although it sounds like a lot, this amount is well tolerated by almost everyone. Since the guinea pig study was done, no other studies in animals or humans on megadoses of vitamin C and osteoarthritis have been reported in the scientific literature.

Why? Vitamin C is inexpensive, safe, and readily available—not to mention the test-tube proof that it stimulates synthesis of collagen and proteoglycans. It's too bad more scientific studies haven't been conducted to confirm or deny the exciting possibilities of vitamin C in treating joint disease in humans.

Wounds Heal Faster

■ Nonetheless, vitamin C does some amazing things for body tissues. One is wound healing. Take major surgery, for example. It's well known that surgery temporarily empties vitamin C stores. This is called "biochemical scurvy." Many studies clearly show that doses of one gram or more enhance the healing of minor wounds, reduce inflammation, and improve recovery. The best results are seen in the sickest people, particularly those whose vitamin C stores were somewhat depleted prior to surgery. The routine use of vitamin C before and after surgery is practiced by many surgeons throughout the world.

With skin ulcers, researchers have found that one or two grams of vitamin C taken daily cuts healing time in half, compared to conventional treatments. This is good news to paraplegics and people with "thalassemia" (a blood disorder), who frequently get large, hard-to-heal skin sores that put them at risk for infection.

Another case report: Two healthy graduate students intentionally wounded the inside of their mouths on three separate occasions (I would not recommend this tactic for the general public). They took either a placebo, one gram of vitamin C, or two grams of vitamin C a day, until the wounds were healed. Both vitamin C doses led to complete healing in nine or ten days, compared to eighteen days with the placebo.

Vitamin C doesn't stop there. Perhaps its best-studied healing effect is in gum disease. With gum disease, there's bone loss, erosion of connective tissue around teeth, and poor resistance to germs in the mouth. One researcher, Dr. Larry Lytle, administered "saturation" doses of vitamin C, as measured by bowel tolerance, to twenty-one patients with long-standing, sensitive, painful gums resistant to usual dental treatments. The doses averaged three hundred times the RDA. After one day, the doses were reduced over a period of four days. Ten of the twenty-one patients were pain-free, nine others showed improvement, and only two remained the same.

This study suggests that if true saturation with vitamin C is achieved, connective tissue responds favorably. Other studies of gum disease and vitamin C have shown that gums improve with supplementation of one or more grams.

In short, vitamin C is surprisingly understudied. What little information we have indicates that high doses (about four grams a day) can potentially bolster the health of connective tissue. We don't know for sure whether it can prevent or reverse arthritis. Even a slim possibility warrants further investigation. But if you have joint problems now, why wait for studies that might never happen?

Tips for Taking Vitamin C

■ Vitamin C is safe at four-gram doses for almost everyone. Taking one gram four times a day (at breakfast, lunch, dinner, and bedtime) just might make a difference in how you feel. Seek advice from your physician for doses larger than four grams.

I like to put vitamin C powder into my juice in the morning. It mixes easily and tastes good in any juice (I haven't tried prune juice yet, however). A slightly heaping teaspoon each day provides about four or five grams of vitamin C. Effervescent (fizzy) vitamin C powders or tablets are also available.

I prefer a "buffered" product. This is a formulation containing essential minerals such as potassium, calcium, and magnesium. These reduce the acidity of vitamin C.

I don't recommend time-release vitamin C tablets because they tend to discharge the nutrient at the wrong time. Nor do I advise using the chewable vitamin C. It coats your teeth with acid and sugar, which might set the stage for tooth cavities. A new form of vitamin C called Ester-C appears to get into cells faster than regular vitamin C supplements. Even so, the clinical superiority of one vitamin C product over another hasn't yet been demonstrated scientifically. Plus, it's still more cost-effective to take regular vitamin C.

Vitamin E: The Potential Is There

■ Vitamin E has been credited with everything from improving your sex life to extending your natural life. Despite some of its exaggerated claims, research shows that higher-than-RDA levels of vitamin E protect against cancer, heart disease, and other chronic degenerative diseases. At the cellular level, vitamin E safeguards cell membranes from oxidation. It is oxidized instead, attracting and then killing off free radicals.

This important vitamin is actually a family of related compounds produced by plants to protect their oils from oxidation by air. Our bodies can't make vitamin E. Like vitamin C, we have to get it from foods.

Can vitamin E work its nutritional magic for joint problems? The jury is still out, since few studies of vitamin E and connective tissue have been done. Research in test tubes and with animals indicates that high doses of vitamin E keep inflammation in check. Animal studies on vitamin E and arthritis have given mixed results. Dr. Schwartz, who conducted the aforementioned guinea pig studies with vitamin C, found that vitamin E reduced the degradation of guinea-pig cartilage cultures and increased the deposition of proteoglycans in cartilage.

One ray of research hope is vitamin E's effect on osteoarthritis. Researchers in Israel administered vitamin E supplements (six hundred milligrams) to twenty-nine patients with osteoarthritis for ten days. The subjects then took placebos the next ten days. When taking vitamin E, over half the patients had marked reductions in pain. Although they were all using painkillers, the vitamin E group used less drugs. These results suggest vitamin E might protect cartilage in humans.

Taking Vitamin E

■ Not all vitamin Es are created equal. There are natural vitamin E products and synthetic ones. Vitamin E is the only vitamin in which the natural-versus-synthetic choice makes a difference. Natural vitamin E is much better absorbed and utlilized by the body.

Most vitamin E studies use the synthetic type, or never mention what kind is used. Synthetic vitamin E products contain seven types of vitamin E. Only one of the seven is natural vitamin E.

How can you tell what you're buying? Read the label. Natural vitamin E contains d-alpha-tocopherol or mixed tocopherols. Less desirable but still useful forms of vitamin E are d-alpha-tocopherol acetate or d-alpha-tocopherol succinate. The least effective synthetic forms of vitamin E begin with a "dl" or "DL" designation. Synthetic vitamin E is half the cost of the real stuff, which is why many supplement manufacturers use it.

Daily doses of natural vitamin E are safe at the four hundred to eight-hundred-IU level. Even higher doses (sixteen hundred IUs) appear safe for most people. Yet these are wasted and might thin the blood in susceptible people. As for synthetic vitamin E, never exceed four hundred IUs per day.

The Healing Possibilities of Beta Carotene

■ Another antioxidant newsmaker is beta carotene, found in many green and yellow fruits and vegetables. Structurally, beta carotene is two molecules of vitamin A joined together. If vitamin A is in short supply, beta carotene splits in half to make two vitamin A molecules, but only on demand. Thus, there is no chance of vitamin A toxicity from beta carotene.

Beta carotene is a different type of antioxidant because it works best against a high-energy form of oxygen called a "singlet oxygen," which produces free radicals. Beta carotene defuses singlet oxygen before it can do its dirty work.

Little is known about the effects of beta carotene and vitamin A on osteoarthritis and other joint problems, since no clinical studies have been done. Interestingly, it was recently discovered that gold salts (a treatment for rheumatoid arthritis) neutralize singlet oxygen, as does beta carotene. This doesn't mean that high doses of beta carotene can be used instead of gold salts, though. Unlike gold salts, not much beta carotene gets to the joints where it can do any good.

Don't discount this antioxidant, however. We now know that antioxidants—vitamin C and vitamin E included—have a "synergistic" effect. That's another way of saying "united we stand, divided we fall." Working together, they're a formidable fighting force against free radicals; alone, they're not as strong. Maybe that's why Mother Nature put beta carotene in foods rich in vitamin C and other antioxidants.

Beta carotene is safe. If you take a lot of it, the palms of your hand and soles of your feet can turn orange. This is beta carotene being stored in your fat cells, and is perfectly harmless.

Vitamin A is a different story. It's toxic taken in large doses. Early Arctic explorers learned this the hard way when they shot and ate polar bears to keep from starving. They didn't know that polar bear livers store a huge amount of vitamin A. Many of the explorers got sick, and some died from too much vitamin A, as well as from exposure to the cold.

A safe dose of beta carotene being suggested by many antioxidant researchers is twenty-five thousand IU daily, and doses of one hundred thousand IU daily have been used medically.

The Selenium/Arthritis Link

■ Selenium is a trace mineral with a specialized function. It activates one of the most important antioxidants in the body: an enzyme called glutathione peroxidase, or GPx (GLUE-ta-THIGH-own per-OX-id-ace). GPx is a biochemical jack-of-all-trades. It uses a molecule called glutathione to get rid of free radicals and repairs their damage. It recharges other antioxidants (vitamin C and vitamin E). And it detoxifies harmful, disease-causing compounds.

Your cells make glutathione from a common amino acid called cysteine. Just to show you how powerful the GPx/glutathione/selenium team is: A form of cysteine is now being used in clinical trials with AIDS patients and producing some benefits.

There's an apparent link between selenium and arthritis. Investigators have found that osteoarthritis sufferers have low levels of selenium in their blood. Deficiencies might even cause arthritis. Areas of the world with a low selenium content in the soil have a higher rate of osteoarthritis, cancer, and heart disease. In parts of China where soil levels of selenium are low, many teenagers have a disabling form of osteoarthritis called Kashin-Beck Disease (KBD). Finland is a selenium-deficient country, too. The law there requires that fertilizers for growing foods and livestock be supplemented with selenium. Since the law was enacted, Finnish people have had less heart disease, cancer, and arthritis.

Does selenium supplementation do any good? Studies have found that it helps relieve pain in some people, but not in everyone. Most of the research exploring osteoarthritis and selenium has found little evidence to support supplementation. These studies, however, used modest amounts of selenium and its antioxidant partners.

Even if selenium did nothing for osteoarthritis, it might still be a good idea to take it—in moderate amounts (up to two hundred fifty micrograms daily)—since the mineral is an important member of the antioxidant family and appears to have a protective effect on the body. Be careful not to take too much, however. It can be toxic. Doses of two hundred fifty micrograms seem safe for everyone.

Other Amazing Antioxidants

■ Other lesser-known antioxidants have surfaced as potential contenders in the fight against joint problems. One is an enzyme called superoxide dismutase (SOD), purified and sold as an injectable drug. When injected into arthritic joints, SOD reduces pain and swelling significantly and improves joint mobility in both osteoarthritis and rheumatoid arthritis patients. Compliance with the treatment is a problem, however, since you have to have a shot. Veterinarians use SOD (called Palosein) to help degenerative joint diseases in animals.

You can buy SOD supplements in health-food stores and from mail-order vitamin companies. But a word of caution: Because SOD is an enzyme, the body digests it like food. So it doesn't really have the same effect as its injectable preparation.

To prevent deficiencies of SOD, make sure you're getting ample amounts of zinc, copper, and manganese in your diet. These minerals activate SOD. A multiple vitamin/mineral supplement is a good safeguard against deficiencies.

One antioxidant that shows some promise is a class of nutrients known as bioflavonoids. Citrus fruits, green and black teas, coffee, green, leafy vegetables, and onion skins are rich sources. Certain bioflavonoids have been isolated and tested for their effects on joints. Some good news: Bioflavonoids seem to protect cultured cartilage tissue from the onslaught of free radicals. Plus, bioflavonoids show some anti-inflammatory activity and seem to preserve vitamin C in the body.

But the downside is that it's difficult to absorb bioflavonoids and get them into the joints. More work is needed to make the promise of bioflavonoids become reality.

If you've ever enjoyed chicken curry, you've eaten a potent antioxidant called curcumin, known to help prevent cancer and heart disease. Curcumin is a compound of turmeric, found in curry spice.

Curcumin is an effective anti-inflammatory, and research bears this out. In a study in India, nineteen people with rheumatoid arthritis were divided into two groups. One group took twelve hundred milligrams of curcumin a day; the other, three hundred milligrams of an NSAID (phenylbutazone). After an unspecified period of time, the protocol was reversed. The results showed that curcumin's anti-inflammatory effect matched that of the drug. Yet phenylbutazone was better at pain relief. Other research has produced similar findings. Curcumin as an anti-inflammatory deserves further study since it is safer than anti-inflammatory drugs.

One antioxidant that shows some promise is a class of nutrients known as bioflavonoids.

An antioxidant increasing in popularity is Pycnogenol. Widely used in France, Pycnogenol is made from a type of pine bark. There are plenty of claims about its effectiveness on degenerative joint disease, but to date no well-designed studies have borne this out. Pycnogenol is expensive, too, so you might want to stick with the basic antioxidants.

ANTIOXIDANTS USED BY OUR CELLS

Vitamins:

    Beta carotene

    Vitamin C (ascorbate)

    Vitamin E (tocopherol)

Minerals:

    Selenium

    Zinc

Enzymes:

    Glutathione Peroxidase (GPx)

    Superoxide Dismutase (SOD)

    Catalase

Amino Acids:

    Glutathione

    L-Cysteine

    L-Methionine

    Taurine

TABLE 6.1

HOW TO USE ANTIOXIDANTS: SAFE DAILY DOSES
OF SUPPLEMENTAL ANTIOXIDANT NUTRIENTS

Antioxidant	Daily Dose
Beta carotene	25,000 to 250,000 IU
Vitamin C (Mineral ascorbates, ascorbic acid)	1,000 to 4,000 mg
Vitamin E (d-alpha-tocopherol or mixed tocopherols)	400 to 800 IU (mg)
Selenium (selenite, selenomethionine or a mixture)	100 to 250 mcg
Cysteine (N-Acetyl-L-Cysteine or NAC)	500 to 2,000 mg

NOTE: The doses listed above are total daily doses. Split the total dose into two or three amounts taken with meals. The best types of each antioxidant are listed below each name. Look for the specific wording mentioned on a product label. If the label wording is not like what is listed in this table, be very suspicious about what you are getting. Ask sales personnel for more information. If buying mail order, don't buy until you are sure of what you're getting.

Other antioxidants, which are optional, include: coenzyme Q10 (ubiquinone); bioflavonoids (green tea catechins, quercetin, citrus source, hesperidin, rutin, silymarins); curcumin; L-methionine; taurine; garlic; proanthocyanidins (Pycnogenol); ferulic acid; gamma oryzanol; and certain herbs like Gingko biloba, Rosemary, Sage, and Thyme. While these antioxidants may have some additional benefits when used along with the nutrient antioxidants listed in the Table, their true value in degenerative joint conditions or joint injuries is not well known at this time. They all appear to be quite safe. It is up to you to determine if possible benefit outweighs the known cost.

TABLE 6.2

7

※━

Second-Line Nutrients
for Arthritis

Picture this scenario: A sixty-year-old man has osteoarthritis so bad that at times he can barely move his joints through a full range of motion. The usual prognosis is bleak: a gradual downhill slide, with no hope for a cure. In all likelihood, the patient is facing long-term drug therapy and a lifetime of pain. Then his doctor steps in and prescribes a B-complex vitamin (niacinamide) to be taken eight times a day. Within a year, there's a dramatic turnaround. He regains most of his joint movement and starts feeling better than he has in years. This patient gets a new lease on life.

A new lease on life? That's the promise of several other nutrients—vitamins, minerals, and special fats—whose therapeutic results are often as dramatic as those of the latest wonder drug. Let's fast forward to a closer look at how doctors and patients are using eight special nutrients to win reprieves from osteoarthritis.

Niacinamide (Vitamin B₃) for Arthritis

■ A now-retired physician from North Carolina, Dr. William Kaufman, M.D., Ph.D., devoted his entire career to studying joint problems and treating them with niacinamide. A member of the

B-complex family, niacinamide plays a role in cellular energy production. Dr. Kaufman published much of his work in a book titled *The Common Form of Joint Dysfunction: Its Incidence and Treatment* in 1949 and continued to document his findings in articles as recently as 1983.

Dr. Kaufman's search for an alternative to the complications of drug therapy began in the forties, a time when deficiency diseases were severe and widespread. One of these was pellagra, a life-threatening illness stemming from a shortage of niacinamide in the diet. Shortly after World War II, refined flour was fortified with vitamins and iron to stave off these diseases. Dr. Kaufman observed that even though the severe symptoms of pellagra disappeared after food fortification, some of the less serious ones remained, among them impaired balance, lack of joint mobility, and muscular weakness.

Dr. Kaufman started prescribing niacinamide to patients with these symptoms and recorded their progress. Within four weeks, their joint mobility improved dramatically. For the next twenty years, Dr. Kaufman kept meticulous records of 663 patients taking niacinamide and 179 patients not taking the vitamin. The patients, who ranged in age from four to eighty years old, had varying degrees of osteoarthritis, rheumatoid arthritis, or both.

The use of niacinamide made a huge difference in more than 70 percent of the patients. The typical pattern of recovery was rapid improvement within a month, followed by slow, steady improvement in joint mobility for two to three years. After that, no further improvements were seen. People with a history of joint problems improved so much that their joint health was better than that of healthy controls their own age!

How is it that niacinamide can have such an impact? We don't exactly know. Niacinamide has no painkilling properties. Nor is it an anti-inflammatory. Even so, joint pain gradually subsided and eventually disappeared in most of these patients. This pattern co-incided with the slow rate of cartilage repair. Somehow, cartilage was fixed, and pain stopped as a result.

Dr. Kaufman applied his knowledge of pharmacology to determine the most effective way to prescribe niacinamide. He knew that giving a supplement of niacinamide increases blood levels of the nutrient for four to six hours. He also knew that blood levels become saturated by a 250-milligram dose. Higher doses are simply wasted. That being the case, he administered one hundred fifty to two hundred fifty milligrams of niacinamide every one to three hours for six to sixteen total doses a day, depending on the severity of the joint problem. Saturating the blood with niacinamide ensures that other tissues, including cartilage, become saturated as well.

Niacinamide isn't a one-time "cure." If you use it for joint problems, you're going to need it long-term. When niacinamide supplementation was stopped, Dr. Kaufman found that joint mobility got worse, and patients returned to their original condition in a matter of weeks. For niacinamide to work, the implication is that supplementation should be continued for a long time. Dr. Kaufman also tried other B vitamins, vitamin B_{12} injections, and vitamins A, C, and D. But none had any effect on joint problems. Dr. Kaufman, however, did not use the high doses of vitamin C described in the previous chapter.

In several thousand "patient-years" of high-dose niacinamide therapy, as well as more than forty years of clinical experience, no adverse side effects were reported or observed. This confirms the findings of the FDA and other expert nutrition panels: Niacinamide is safe.

A word of warning, though: Don't confuse niacinamide with niacin. Both are vitamin B_3, but niacin acts in a completely different manner. At high doses, niacin has unpleasant, potentially damaging side effects, including flushing; bright-red rashes on the face, neck, and arms; and severe tingling or itching. In a worst-case scenario, high doses can damage the liver. Niacin is used as a drug to lower blood cholesterol levels and should be taken only under a doctor's supervision.

Both niacin and niacinamide improve joint function. But because of niacin's drawbacks, only niacinamide should be used. Always consult your physician before starting on high-dose niacinamide therapy.

Only one other investigator, Dr. Abram Hoffer, a Canadian psychiatrist and researcher, has confirmed Dr. Kaufman's results. Using high-dose niacin or niacinamide therapy for other medical conditions, Dr. Hoffer found that his patients with arthritis improved unexpectedly, in the same time intervals as Dr. Kaufman's patients.

Why Dr. Kaufman's amazing results have not been investigated and repeated by other researchers is a great mystery. The sheer longevity of his work, the objective measurements, and the known role of niacinamide at the cellular level make a strong argument for further clinical research.

Pyridoxine (Vitamin B$_6$) and Carpal Tunnel Syndrome

■ It starts with a numbness in all your fingers, except in your pinky. Pain from your wrist shoots up into your forearm. At night, you wake up hurting so much that you want to scream.

The diagnosis? Carpal tunnel syndrome. It's a swelling, or inflammation, of a passageway through the wrists called the carpal tunnel, which protects nerves and ligaments that extend into your hand. The nerves get squeezed, producing pain, numbness, and muscle weakness. In some cases, carpal tunnel syndrome is so severe that hand function can be temporarily lost. People who use their hands repetitively in their jobs—typists, carpenters, store clerks, mechanics, and others—often get carpal tunnel syndrome. The treatment? Resting the joint, wearing a wrist splint, taking injectable steroids, having surgery—or supplementing with vitamin B_6.

Otherwise known as pyridoxine, vitamin B_6 is important for protein and fat metabolism, as well as for blood formation. It has been widely studied as a treatment for carpal tunnel syndrome. But the reviews are mixed.

Carpal tunnel patients who respond best to vitamin B_6 therapy are those with a hidden or obvious deficiency of the vitamin. They need no other treatment. Patients without a deficiency seldom benefit from taking vitamin B_6, according to studies. Even so, medical experts now recommend supplementing with vitamin B_6 (one hundred milligrams daily, plus fifty milligrams daily of vitamin B_2) for three months. If there's no let-up of symptoms, then the patient becomes a candidate for surgery.

Some guidelines on taking vitamin B_6: Don't exceed one hundred milligrams a day. This is a safe dose; higher doses can be toxic. Upon exposure to air, a tiny amount of vitamin B_6 becomes oxidized (damaged), converting it into anti-vitamin B_6. With someone taking very large amounts of vitamin B_6, the oxidized form builds up, eventually reaching significant levels. The anti-vitamin turns into a "bad guy" vitamin that knocks out the remaining "good" vitamin B_6. Your body thinks there's a shortage as a result.

> *People who use their hands repetitively in their jobs—typists, carpenters, store clerks, mechanics, and others—often get carpal tunnel syndrome.*

A newly available form of vitamin B_6 is now on the market: pyridoxal-5-phosphate or B_6 phosphate. This is a purer form of the nutrient, the same type that's found in foods, so there is less chance of oxidized vitamin B_6 forming.

If you've been diagnosed with carpal tunnel syndrome, it's worth trying vitamin B_6 for three months. If nothing happens and the pain persists, there may be no way short of surgery to make carpal tunnel syndrome go away.

Magnesium for Joint Health

■ For a long time, magnesium was the Rodney Dangerfield of minerals: It got no respect. Now that's changing. Magnesium is known to be involved in all cellular process, as well as in all aspects of joint maintenance and repair. New studies suggest that our society as a whole might fall short of the magnesium needed for good health. Women, in particular, are at risk. National surveys by government agencies have found that about half of all American women might be magnesium-deficient.

How do you know if you're getting enough of this precious mineral (three hundred fifty to four hundred milligrams a day)? Some bodily responses to a deficiency are fatigue, muscle spasms, grinding teeth at night, depression, anxiety, confusion, nervousness, loss of appetite, bloating, and insomnia.

One of magnesium's critical roles is in bone mass. In fact, it might be as important as calcium in maintaining healthy bones. A research case in point: Giving magnesium supplements, along with calcium, promoted bone mass by up to 11 percent in one year in women with bone loss.

Findings like this are important for degenerative joint disease. As described earlier, a feature of osteoarthritis is bone remodeling (osteophyte formation), the dissolution and rebuilding of bone around arthritic joints. Theoretically, a good supply of magne-sium will let bone remodel more normally, with less bone thick-ening. This could potentially help ease the pain of osteoarthritis.

Many physicians are already using magnesium with arthritis patients to help improve overall health, including joint health. We don't know yet whether magnesium will reverse osteoarthritis. But this much is certain: A magnesium deficiency can make arthritis worse.

Magnesium is found in whole grains, green, leafy vegetables, beans, and nuts. The surest way to make certain you're getting enough is by supplementing your diet with magnesium. Daily doses of between two hundred and four hundred milligrams are enough to shore up your supply of magnesium. The "best" forms of magnesium supplements are:

- ◆ magnesium glycinate
- ◆ magnesium citrate
- ◆ magnesium aspartate
- ◆ magnesium chloride
- ◆ magnesium lactate
- ◆ magnesium orotate
- ◆ magnesium chelates with branched-chain amino acids.

Other types might not be absorbed as well. The magnesium found in antacid products is not a good dietary source of the mineral.

Cartilage-Making Manganese

■ Manganese is an obscure mineral, although not when it comes to joint health. Its main role in the body is to activate the enzymes needed to make cartilage. A shortfall of manganese can cause arthritis, joint degeneration, and bone loss.

No one knows how serious manganese deficiencies really are. In certain parts of Africa, the content of manganese in the soil is low. The inhabitants there frequently get Mseleni disease, a severe form of osteoarthritis.

There's a link between age-related bone and cartilage loss and the amount of manganese you have in cartilage tissue. Studies show that the older you get, the less manganese you have in your cartilage. Some research suggests that manganese might help prevent or reverse osteoporosis; however, there's no similar information on using manganese supplements for osteoarthritis. Given the alarming rate of osteoarthritis, the connection between it and manganese deserves more attention.

Manganese is plentiful in whole grains, nuts, legumes, and fresh vegetables and fruit. Eating meat with manganese-rich foods helps your body better absorb the mineral.

If you've been diagnosed as having bone or cartilage loss, consider manganese supplementation. The best forms include:

- ◆ manganese ascorbate
- ◆ manganese gluconate
- ◆ other amino acid chelates

Poorly absorbed forms are manganese sulfate and manganese oxide. A daily dose of five to fifty milligrams is both safe and adequate.

Copper: A Potential Anti-Arthritic Agent

■ Perhaps your grandmother claimed that drinking apple cider made in copper-lined kettles tamed her creaky hip. Or your Aunt Mary wore a copper bracelet to keep her rheumatism from acting up.

Copper as a cure for arthritis is deeply rooted in folk medicine tradition. Could your relatives have been right? Is there any credence in the copper remedy?

Possibly. But not for apple cider "cures." There's no truth to the tale, say the scientists who studied it, maybe because the cider wasn't cooked up in copper kettles.

Copper bracelets and other copper devices, however, have stood up to the test. Wearers with rheumatoid arthritis do feel some relief, according to scientific studies. In fact, pharmaceutical companies have synthesized and isolated hundreds of copper compounds. Today, some of these copper compounds are being studied in animals as potential anti-arthritis treatments—and showing promise. Also, D-penicillamine, a drug used to treat rheumatoid arthritis, is now believed to work by interacting with copper. Proof is piling up that copper may be helpful in rheumatic diseases.

What about osteoarthritis? Right now, there's not much evidence to show that taking copper over and above daily requirements does any good. Still, many of us are slightly deficient in copper. National surveys say that we get only half the copper we need in our diets. A shortfall can impair the ability of bone and cartilage to heal normally.

Because many Americans are copper-deficient, supplementing with copper is a good idea for people with joint problems. A daily dose of two milligrams (the suggested safe and adequate daily dietary intake) is good insurance against a deficiency. The best-absorbed sources are:

- ◆ copper glycinate
- ◆ gluconate
- ◆ histidinate
- ◆ lysinate
- ◆ sebacate

Get in Sync with Zinc

■ Your body needs zinc to make—and repair—every one of its cells. Zinc is in demand for wound and fracture healing, bone metabolism, growth, and pregnancy—any situation where cells are rapidly dividing. Too little zinc can make big trouble, including bone loss and joint damage.

Will taking extra zinc help osteoarthritis? We don't yet know for sure. To date, zinc supplementation has been studied for use in treating rheumatoid and psoriatic arthritis, but not osteoarthritis. Results from eleven well-conducted trials with zinc sulfate (a harsh, toxic salt) have shown benefits in some people, but not in all. Mixed results like these indicate merit, however. Further research is needed, particularly with other more palatable zinc supplements such as zinc methionate, zinc histidinate, zinc picolinate, zinc aspartate, or zinc citrate.

There's evidence that zinc intake is below the RDA for many Americans. Because of its role in bone and soft tissue formation, it's critical to get enough of this mineral. A safe dose for supplementation is fifteen to twenty-five milligrams of zinc a day in one of the forms listed above. This amount is usually found in multiple vitamin/mineral supplement. Don't take a formulation using zinc sulfate or zinc oxide, however. These salts might cause stomach irritation and nausea.

Boron for Bones

■ The trace mineral boron is found in nature as borate, the same compound used in Twenty-Four Mule Team Borax detergent. Boron is known to be involved in many specialized functions, including hormonal activity and the transport of nutrients across cell membranes.

Boron was big news in 1987 when USDA researchers found that older women, fed a boron-deficient diet, started to show the preliminary signs of osteoporosis. When boron (as borate) was fed to the women, their estrogen levels went back up. This study has been misinterpreted as proving that boron raises hormone levels and thus can replace estrogen therapy for osteoporosis. Not true. This study shows that a boron deficiency is bad news for bones. Additional dietary boron does not elevate hormone levels correspondingly. Nevertheless, boron might help prevent osteoporosis.

As for osteoarthritis, some interesting research has emerged. Areas with low boron content in the soil have been linked to high rates of osteoarthritis in the population. In Australia, researchers found that boron supplements helped ease osteoarthritis. They gave six milligrams of boron (as borate) to ten subjects and gave a placebo to ten controls. After eight weeks, five of the ten boron-supplemented subjects and one of the controls felt improvement. The boron group had less joint pain and did not change their pain medication. The control group still experienced pain and had to take even more medication. The findings suggest that boron has a role to play in the treatment of osteoarthritis.

Fresh fruits and vegetables are good sources of boron, but levels depend on the soil in which they were grown.

Fresh fruits and vegetables are good sources of boron, but levels depend on the soil in which they were grown. Interestingly, the soil levels of boron are low in the United States, with a corresponding high rate of osteoarthritis. Getting your daily dose from food might not be so easy. A safe dose is three to six milligrams a day. Boron appears to work in close balance with magnesium, manganese, copper, and zinc. With its apparent benefit in osteoarthritis and degenerative bone disease, boron is one mineral to have on your side.

Fishing For Relief: Omega-3 Fats

■ Unless you've been living on a desert island, you've probably heard about omega-3 fats, found mostly in deep-sea fish. The evidence in favor of their protective effect on health, particularly the immune system, is striking. These polyunsaturated fats are needed to make hormone-like substances called "prostaglandins." Certain prostaglandins known as the "good" type help the immune system do its job–fending off disease, fighting infection, and reducing inflammation.

Because of the prostaglandin connection, fish oils have the potential to act as anti-inflammatory agents. Accordingly, researchers have tested fish oil supplementation in patients with rheumatoid arthritis, with positive results. Patients reported less joint tenderness, reduced stiffness in the morning, and less reliance on anti-inflammatory drugs and pain medication. Plus, researchers found an increase in the activity of good prostaglandins. The effects were moderate, but still significant. The only drawback was that patients had to take ten to fifteen fish oil capsules a day. This dosage caused them to burp up dead-fish smells all day long. There were no other bad side effects, however. You can get omega-3 fats from other non-fish sources. These include flaxseed oil, flaxseeds, and purslane, which is used as a decorative plant in the United States and in salads in Mediterranean cuisine. Canola oil and soybean oil also have traces of omega-3 fats.

As for osteoarthritis, low-back pain, and other joint injuries, no specific studies have looked into the effects of using omega-3s. But since there's mild inflammation associated with osteoarthritis, fish oil might offer some relief.

There's a catch to using omega-3 fats. In Table 7.3, you'll find some dietary changes that make omega-3 fats work better at lower doses. If you eat a high-fat diet (not recommended), you have to intake even more omega-3 fat to get results.

It's puzzling as to why nutrients with known roles in connective-tissue health have been barely studied using people with osteoarthritis, low-back pain, and joint injuries as subjects. The few existing studies show very promising results. Likewise, clinical benefits for other closely related joint problems such as rheumatoid arthritis indicate the health-protective effects of certain nutrients. Knowing which nutrients have an impact on joint health is an important tool in preventing and possibly reversing joint disease.

PROPER USE OF NIACINAMIDE
FOR JOINT DISORDERS

Severity of Joint Disorder	Daily Oral Dosage Sched.	Total Dose (mg)
Slight	150-250 mg every three hours for six doses	900-1,500
Moderate (about 75 percent of normal mobility)	250 mg every three hours for six doses or 250 mg every two hours for eight doses	1,500-2,000
Severe (about half of normal mobility)	250 mg every two hours for eight doses or 250 mg every 1.5 hours for ten doses	2,000-2,500
Extremely severe (less than half of normal mobility)	250 mg every 1.5 hours for ten doses or 250 mg every hour for sixteen doses	2,500-4,000

TABLE 7.1

MINERALS IMPORTANT TO JOINTS:
GUIDELINES FOR USE

Mineral (Desired Forms)	Daily Doses
Magnesium (aspartate, branched-chain amino acid chelate, chloride, citrate, glycinate, lactate, orotate)	200 to 400 mg
Manganese (ascorbate, gluconate)	5 to 50 mg
Copper (glycinate, gluconate, histidinate, lysinate, sebacate)	2 mg
Zinc (aspartate, citrate, histidinate, methionate, picolinate)	15 or 25 mg
Boron (sodium borate)	6 mg

TABLE 7.2

DIETARY CHANGES TO ENHANCE
OMEGA-3 FAT FUNCTIONS

1. Eat a low-fat diet. Preferably, 10 to 15 percent of calories should come from fat.

2. Stop eating foods with high levels of saturated fat. These foods include red meats, dairy products (whole milk, 2-percent milk, ice cream, butter, cheese, cream), margarine, shortening, lard, tallow, chocolate (cocoa butter), and fried foods. Coconut fat is saturated, but is not a problem.

3. Learn how to cook without using extra fat. Do not put butter, margarine, or other oils on foods.

4. Limit intake of most vegetable oils. This includes vegetable cooking oils, corn oil, safflower oil, sunflower oil, soybean oil, sesame oil, peanut oil, nuts, seeds, peanuts, and peanut butter. An ideal intake is one tablespoon per day.

5. Eat more fish, especially fish with colored flesh (salmon, mackerel, sardines, herring, anchovies, tuna, eel). Shellfish and blue-green algae are good sources of omega-3 fats, too. Eat these foods at least once daily.

6. Optional: Add fish oil supplements (not fish liver oil). Three to eighteen capsules are doses used in studies, but each person must find what they can tolerate.

7. Add flaxseed oil (edible linseed oil), one tablespoon daily (or three to nine capsules daily). Flaxseed oil must be kept in the freezer, and can't be used in cooking. It does work in salads. Flaxseed oil may be used in place of fish oil.

8. Increase fresh, green, leafy vegetable consumption. All those green plants have relatively low levels of omega-3 fats, but also contain other healthy nutrients like vitamin C, beta carotene, vitamin E, and minerals.

....

9. Add a vitamin E supplement (d-alpha-tocopherol), 100 or 400 IU per day. This keeps the omega-3 fats from breaking down in your body.

....

10. Optional: Add GLA oil supplements, three capsules daily. GLA oils assist Omega-3 fats to make good prostaglandins. There are even supplements that combine Omega-3 and GLA oils. GLA oils include evening primrose, blackcurrant seed, and borage seed oils.

....

TABLE 7.3

8

Supplements That Accelerate Healing

You use them every time you clean your contact lenses or sprinkle meat tenderizer on a piece of beef. They were once prescription drugs used successfully to treat inflammation, before the synthetic painkillers came on the scene. Yet few people have ever heard of them.

They're called "proteases," enzyme nutrients found in all living things. In supplemental form, they might be one of your best bets for relief from joint problems and sports injuries. Two of the most common proteases come from fruits: bromelain from pineapples and papain from papayas.

Just what are proteases, and how do they work? Let's find out.

The Healing Power of Proteases

■ Proteases are enzymes that chew up protein. They're at work in digestion, cell division, cell replacement, immune function, and more. Your body has its own team of proteases that travel to injured sites to control inflammation and promote healing. Supplemental proteases are backups that help natural proteases do their job better.

The clinical evidence in support of protease supplementation is encouraging. For example:

◆ Amateur boxers in England who supplemented with proteases healed their bruises and cuts twice as fast as those
who took placebos (five days versus two weeks). Taking
proteases before boxing matches worked even better than
taking them afterward.

◆ Athletes at the University of Delaware using protease supplements were able to cut their recovery time from athletic injuries from 8.4 days to 3.9 days. At the University of
Pittsburgh, football players given proteases found that
minor injuries healed faster, compared to the injuries of
placebo-treated players.

◆ The knee is one of the most-injured parts of the body in
athletics. When a group of knee-surgery patients in
Germany were given proteases, they could bend their
knees a full 90 degrees seven days after surgery. For those
on placebos, it took nine days.

◆ Taking proteases cuts down on hospital stays. After
surgery for fractures, patients supplemented with proteases left the hospital after 17.7 days, compared to 24.1 days
for placebo-treated patients.

◆ When forty-four people with severely sprained ankles
supplemented with proteases, they experienced less pain
and swelling, and were able to move around better than
nonsupplemented controls. The protease group returned
to work in 1.7 days, compared to 4.4 days for the controls.

◆ For aching backs, proteases bring relief. At Guy's Hospital
Arthritis Research Unit in London, ninety-three patients
were given proteases for low-back pain. The results were
promising: Pain and inflammation subsided so much that
their dosage of painkillers was cut. Leg-mobility problems,

often a complication of low-back pain, improved significantly. A closer look into these results revealed that proteases actually reduced inflammation around nerve endings compressed by herniated discs or bony overgrowths in the spine. Although proteases didn't cure low-back pain, they did alleviate some symptoms.

◆ In several studies involving patients with injuries, 90 percent of the subjects had less pain, swelling, and redness after taking protease supplements. Plus, they healed faster and returned to productive living sooner.

◆ Proteases have been used successfully to reduce pain, reduce swelling, and speed recovery from obstetrical surgery, hand-fracture surgery, vasectomies, plastic surgery, dental surgery, tooth extractions, vein stripping, and many other minor surgeries.

Hundreds more credible scientific studies and articles have documented that proteases are beneficial for bruises, sprains, strains, fractures, low-back pain, post-surgical healing, digestive problems, and thrombosis, among others. Not only that, the more severe or chronic the condition, the more effective proteases are. The major proteases found as nutritional supplements are listed in Table 8.1 on (page 119)

A Natural Anti-Inflammatory

■ One summer, I decided to test the anti-inflammatory powers of proteases on myself. Yardwork in my hometown of Houston, Texas, always gives me a mild sunburn on my shoulders. I turn red, then brown, and finally I peel—all in a week's time. Sunburn produces inflammation on one of the largest organs in your body—the skin.

This particular time, I took proteases *before* doing yardwork, *during* it, and *afterward* for three days. The first day, as usual, I turned red. The next day, the redness was gone. In its place was a brown tan, which before would show up after two days. The tan disappeared in three days, and I never peeled. I'm convinced that proteases reduced my inflammation and sped up my sunburn healing process by two or three days. However, don't try this at home! Nor should you expect proteases to rescue you from staying out in the sun too long.

Taking Proteases Successfully

■ In studies by pharmaceutical companies, proteases are well documented for their anti-inflammatory action in acute injuries. They are true anti-inflammatory agents, but without the side effects of NSAIDs. Proteases are also safe, and the proof is in the forty-plus years of use by millions of people. Keep in mind that proteases might not work well for chronic conditions such as osteoarthritis.

Although proteases reduce pain, they don't stop it cold, as do aspirin, prescription drugs, and other painkillers. To some, the pain reduction will be mild; to others, dramatic. It all depends on your pain threshold.

Regardless of their effects on pain, proteases do something conventional anti-inflammatory drugs don't: They enhance the healing process. I consider them one of the best nutrient-healers for severe injuries, including joint injuries.

To get the best results from protease supplementation, here are some guidelines to follow:

◆ Start supplementing as soon after an injury as you can. Better yet, take protease supplements one or two hours before a game, match, or surgery. Proteases don't work well if an injury is three or more days old.

◆ Take five to ten tablets at a time, depending on the size of the tablets. Take ten if the tablets are small; five, if large. (A large tablet is one that can only be swallowed one at a time.)

◆ For best results, take protease supplements on an empty stomach with water or juice, but not milk (it will interfere with protease activity and absorption).

◆ Take protease supplements four times a day, about thirty minutes before meals and before bedtime.

◆ Continue this schedule seven days or until healing has occurred. If there are no results in seven days, they won't happen later.

◆ Select a protease product that is "enteric-coated" (to resist stomach acid) and is formulated with more than one type of protease enzyme. The more proteases listed, the better. Combinations of trypsin, chymotrypsin, bromelain, and papain are best. So are fungal proteases.

There's lots of variation in the potency of enzymes used in commercial protease supplements, so choosing the best product is difficult. I've analyzed dozens of these products and have found that many had little or no activity. Others, however, had more activity than even prescription protease products. My advice: Try various products until you find one that works. Then stick with it.

Anti-Inflammatory Merit in Old-Time Cures

■ Got joint pain? Then chew on some willow bark or rub some red pepper on your joint.

In a bygone era, such folk remedies did spell relief. Willow bark contains salicin, a pain-killer used for thousands of years to treat headaches, rheumatism, and fever. Salicin was later modified and synthesized into what we today know as aspirin. The active ingredient in red pepper is capsaicin, used today in many commercial muscle rubs to relieve aches and pains.

About one-third of all modern medicines come from herbs and plants. Even so, distrust of commercial drugs and fear of side effects have sent some people to their spice rack or health-food store, searching for an herbal cure.

About one-third of all modern medicines come from herbs and plants.

Some herbal remedies may work. Many studies in animals and cell cultures have demonstrated that certain herbs do have anti-inflammatory properties. But studies with humans are seriously lacking.

Just because herbs are natural doesn't mean they're safe. A major problem is quality control. Legally, herbs are classified as foods or as food supplements, and therefore not subject to the same regulations as drugs. You really don't know what you're getting—how it was grown and processed, and whether there are differences in potency from batch to batch. Some herbs are known toxins. Then there's the question of the best way to take it—as a tea, in an extract or tincture, or in a pill.

Using herbs to treat degenerative joint disease is still more folklore than science. That makes it difficult to predict what to expect from using herbal remedies off the shelf. If you use herbs at all, do so in conjunction with your medical treatment. Table 8.3 lists herbs known to have some anti-inflammatory effect.

MAJOR PROTEASES FOUND
IN SUPPLEMENT PRODUCTS

Enzyme	Source
Bromelain	Pineapple
Papain	Papaya
Fungal ("vegetarian") Proteases	Aspergillus molds
Trypsin/chymotrypsin	Hog pancreas
Pancreatin	Hog pancreas

Guidelines for Proper Use:

1. Start supplementation as soon as possible after injury occurs. Taking proteases before an event is even better.

2. Take five to ten tablets four times daily on an empty stomach (very important). Water or juice is preferred to take tablets. The easiest way is to take tablets thirty minutes before each meal and bedtime. If tablets are large, take five at a time. If tablets are small, take ten at a time.

3. Enteric coated tablets are preferred.

4. Multiple proteases are preferred. Read the labels. Combinations of trypsin, chymotrypsin, bromelain, and papain are best. Fungal proteases are also effective.

5. Continue supplementation until healed or for one week, then stop.

TABLE 8.1

WHEN TO SUPPLEMENT WITH ORAL PROTEASES

Acute, Traumatic Injuries:

Bruises, hematomas, contusions, ecchymoses

Sprains, stretched ligaments

Strains, muscle pulls, charley horses

Cuts, lacerations, wounds, abrasions

Fractures

Surgical procedures of all kinds (check with surgeon first)

Chronic Conditions:

Acute low-back pain, sciatica

Bursitis, tendinitis, tenosynovitis, metatarsalgia

Rheumatoid arthritis flare-ups

Prophylactic Use
(take ahead of time for sports with high risk of injury):

Minor surgeries, football games, wrestling matches, soccer games, hockey games, basketball games, rugby games, lacrosse games, rodeo events, car racing, martial arts training, boxing matches, American Gladiator competition

TABLE 8.2

HERBS WITH POTENTIAL
ANTI-INFLAMMATORY EFFECTS

Angelica (Angelica archangelica)

Aloe (Aloe vera)

Arnica (Arnica montana)

Ashwagandha, Indian Ginseng (Withania somnifera)

Birch (Betula pendula)

Black Cohosh (Cimicifuga racemosa)

Blue Cohosh (Caulophyllum thalictroides)

Boswellia (Boswellia serrata)

Chaparral (Larrea tridentata)

Comfrey (Symphytum officinale)

Devil's Claw (Harpagophytum procumbens)

Feverfew (Tanacetum chrysanthemum)

Green Tea (Camelia sinensis)

Guggal (Commiphora mukul)

Khat (Catha edulis)

Licorice (Glycyrrhiza glabra)

Meadowsweet (Filipendula ulmaria)

Turmeric (Curcuma longa)

White Poplar (Populus tremuloides)

Wild Celery Seed (Apium graveolens)

Wild Yam (Dioscorea villosa)

Willow Bark (Salix alba)

Wintergreen (Gaultheria procumbens)

Wormwood (Artemisia absinthium)

Sources:

Agents-Actions. *Supplement 27* (1989). 231-283.

Duke, J.A. *Handbook of Medicinal Herbs.* Boca Raton, Florida: CRC Press, 1985.

Mowrey, D.B. *The Scientific Validation of Herbal Medicine.* 1986.

Weiss, R.F. *Herbal Medicine.* Gothenburg, Sweden: AB Arcanum, 1988.

TABLE 8.3

PART THREE

Nutritional Protocols for Joint Health

9

Dietary Support for Your Joints

Eating right is simply a matter of getting back to nature. A good rule of thumb is to eat foods that are as close to their natural state as possible. This is what our bodies are designed to do. You should be eating a bowl of blueberries, not a blueberry-flavored Pop Tart; a bowl of strawberries, not strawberry shortcake; baked potatoes, not reconstituted mashed potatoes; a real apple, not applesauce; crisp, fresh, raw vegetables, not their canned counterparts; a fish fillet, not fish sticks.

Forget about junk foods or processed foods. Stick with real foods.

This advice is not new, and is being expounded by major organizations such as the U.S. government, American Heart Association, American Dietetics Association, and the National Cancer Institute. As you can see, eating right leads to good health, no matter what part of the body you are visualizing. Healthy eating helps the cardiovascular system, prevents cancer, prevents obesity, and yes, helps maintain healthy joints.

This chapter gives broad guidelines about how to eat for your joints, with advice that also spills over to every other part of your body. This topic alone is the subject of numerous books, and it is *not* the intent of this book to be another diet book. Remember, the studies mentioned in previous chapters did not control their subjects' diets. In other words, the results were seen without a change from dietary habits that were most likely not very good. Imagine what kind of results could be obtained if a healthy diet was also fed. This is where you can stack the nutritional odds in your favor.

Bad Fat Might Be Your Biggest Foe

■ When it comes to bad fats, saturated fat—the kind that's solid at room temperature—wears the blackest hat of all. It's a major culprit in a whole range of diseases, including heart disease, cancer, and obesity. You can now add joint disease to the list.

When it comes to bad fats, saturated fat—the kind that's solid at room temperature—wears the blackest hat of all.

More than thirty years ago, scientists discovered that saturated fats were bad for joints. Back then, scientists used to believe that simply being overweight caused or worsened osteoarthritis.

This theory was put to the test. Researchers selected a strain of mice known to develop osteoarthritis on their own, without any interventions. Large numbers of these mice were put on special diets before they became arthritic. Mice in one group were overfed with lard (a food rich in saturated fats) until they became obese. Mice in another group were overfed with polyunsaturated fat (vegetable oil) until they, too, became equally obese. Mice in a control group were fed a regular mouse diet, and they remained lean and non-obese.

The saturated-fat mice developed more osteoarthritis than the lean controls or the vegetable-fat mice. In fact, the vegetable-fat mice had no more osteoarthritis than the lean mice.

This study clearly showed that saturated fat harmed the joints. Just being overweight was not a primary cause of osteoarthritis.

How do saturated fats hurt joints? The answer might lie in prostaglandins. As you might recall, prostaglandins (eicosanoids) are powerful regulators of cell function, produced from specific polyunsaturated fats. There are "good" and "bad" prostaglandins. Good prostaglandins reduce pain and inflammation; bad ones increase these symptoms. Some of each are necessary to sustain life. In osteoarthritis, an overabundance of bad prostaglandins is produced in joints. Bad prostaglandins are made by cells from fats found in foods high in saturated fats, while good prostaglandins are made from healthier fats such as omega-3 fats found in fish, flaxseed oil, and green, leafy vegetables. Thus, saturated fats themselves are a marker for foods with bad fats.

Bad fats are found in dairy products, most red meat, shortenings, margarines, and partially hydrogenated oils. Since Americans have been eating foods high in saturated fats for most of this century, it is little wonder that degenerative joint disease is rampant. Just like the mice eating too much lard, many Americans have been eating themselves into osteoarthritis.

Saturated fat is a nonessential nutrient. You can live without eating any saturated fat. In fact, you might live longer and be more healthy if you don't eat saturated fat. Your body will make all the saturated fat it needs from sugar, carbohydrates, protein, or other fats.

In fact, any excess amount of sugar, from sweets or starches, will be easily converted by your body's mechanisms into saturated fat. Foods high in sugar are almost never close to their natural state. Foods high in refined starches (like white flour) are quickly and efficiently converted into glucose (blood sugar) by metabolism. It is quite easy to get excess sugar and, therefore, force your body to make even more saturated fat. Yes, go easy on sugar-laden foods.

How to Eat for Healthy Joints

■ Table 9.1 (page 131) lists general dietary guidelines that you should ask yourself every time you sit down to eat. Am I eating any junk foods? Am I eating any fresh, raw fruits, or vegetables? Am I eating food cooked in fat? Am I putting a high-fat condiment (butter, margarine, cream, cheese spread, mayonnaise, bacon bits) on my food? Make your answers fit the yes guidelines.

Tables 9.2 (page 132) and 9.3 (page 134) give sample daily menus. There is actually a tremendous variety of healthy foods. Many do not require a lot of preparation time. You might need to alter your shopping and cooking habits, but the change is well worth the effort. If you want to be healthier, the most important thing you can do is control what you put in your mouth. You are in charge. Put healthy foods in the mouth, not the usual junk.

The healthy sample menus are compared to a bad daily menu. If the bad daily menu looks like your diet, please change!

Comparing Good and Bad Diets

■ To give you an idea of how you can dramatically alter your diet in favor of supporting joint health, just look at a comparison of the three sample daily menus (listed in Table 9.3).

As you can see, the first sample menu, containing meat, is a relatively low-calorie diet at 1,420 calories daily. The total percentage of fat is 26 percent, which is boosted by adding two tablespoons of flaxseed oil daily. Flaxseed oil is half omega-3 fat, a very rich dietary source. Combined with fish, this menu supplies the highest amount of omega-3 fat, even at lower calories. This means that most of those twenty-two grams of polyunsaturated fat are omega-3 fats, which we have previously discussed as being healthy for joints, and making good prostaglandins. The saturated-fat content is very low at eight grams a day. Also, sodium content is low, unless one chooses condiments high in salt. However, even with low-fat, healthy eating, possible deficiencies of calcium, zinc, and copper are apparent. This can be easily corrected by adding one or two glasses of skim milk daily.

The healthy vegetarian diet weighs in at two thousand calories a day, which is close to the proper amount for most people. As you can see, by using nonfat dairy products, there is plenty of protein, and absolutely no deficiencies of any essential nutrient. This particular diet will have less in the way of omega-3 fats than the meat-containing diet. Most of the omega-3 fats come from flaxseed oil and walnuts. Some fresh nuts (walnuts, hazelnuts, chestnuts) are good dietary sources of omega-3 fats. So you can see that eating enough calories to be well fed really can be healthy, even without meat.

Now we get to a typical American daily menu (the bad menu). Notice the slightly higher calories. This is why many Americans are overweight, but can't understand why. Fat is hidden in many convenient foods we are accustomed to eating. Even worse, the Wholeness Index, a measure of how close to its natural state each food is, shows only a 50-percent reading. Thus, half of the entire day's diet is not close to its original form. And this is not such a bad daily menu, either, compared to those of some people I know (hopefully not you). We see that there is a high amount of cholesterol, much of which will be damaged by heat and storage. This gets into why we need more antioxidants; to help protect us from rancid fats. Remember that cholesterol is just like a polyunsaturated fat, and is easily attacked and damaged by free radicals and oxygen in the air. Cooking accelerates the process.

The most important point to make about our bad menu is the kinds of fat. Notice that there is a lot of saturated fat (about three times as much as the healthy diets). There is also more monoun-saturated fat. This is not technically bad for you, but it can still overwhelm good polyunsaturated fats when it comes time to make prostaglandins. With all that extra, nonessential fat in the diet (and in the body), it is small wonder that more bad prostaglandins are likely to be formed. The ratio of polyunsatu-rated fats to other fats is completely reversed (wrongly) in the bad menu. This means that even eating less of the bad menu to con-trol calories will still lead to formation of more bad prostaglandins.

Just look at how many nutrients that we now know are vital for joint health are deficient in the bad menu. Even though there is more food and more calories, there is less essential nutrients. This is the importance of eating foods close to their natural state. Processing removes much of the essential micronutrients such as fiber and minerals from previously good foods. Notice that vita-min E and essential minerals are mostly deficient. This spells trouble for already semistarved chondrocytes in cartilage. Eating this way (the typical American diet) will doom your cartilage to never getting enough of the vital minerals it needs to make more glucosamine, more GAGs, more collagen, and more cartilage. It will be very difficult to fully repair joint injuries or reverse de-generative joint disease on this diet.

From many nutritional angles, a typical American diet stacks the deck of playing cards against your joints. Your joints don't have a chance to keep healthy. In time, as injuries or improper lifestyle situations mount, your joints will get further and further from health. Now it is easy to see why there is such a strong link between joint health and nutrition. Our usual diet is a recipe for cartilage disaster, which is exactly what the statistics tell us.

DIETARY GUIDELINES FOR HEALTHY JOINTS

YES

Adequate caloric intake
(16 calories per pound of body weight)

Whole, fresh foods
(fresh fruits and vegetables, whole grains)

Fish, poultry, extra-lean red meat, wild game, eggs, nonfat dairy products (protein sources)

Low-fat cooking methods
(steam, poach, boil, bake, broil, grill, microwave, nonstick cookware)

Low-fat condiments
(nonfat yogurt and mayonnaise, herb seasonings, mustards, salsa)

NO

Junk, refined, processed foods
(donuts, candy, snacks, white flour, sugar)

High-fat foods
(fried, greasy foods, butter, margarine, shortening, partially hydrogenated oils, many cheeses, cream cheese, mayonnaise)

Cheap red meats
(hot dogs, hamburger, lunch meats, bacon, sausages, most pork cuts)

Cooking with saturated fat
(cut out lard, grease, margarine, butter)

TABLE 9.1

HEALTHY SAMPLE DAILY MENU
(CONTAINING MEAT)

BREAKFAST:

Lox (or smoked salmon)

Whole-wheat bagel

Nonfat cream cheese

Juice (orange, grapefruit, apple, cranberry, etc.)

Grapefruit half or melon half or berries

LUNCH:

Tuna salad sandwich

    Canned tuna packed in water with less salt

    Nonfat mayonnaise (or one tablespoon flaxseed oil)

    Diced celery

    Mustard to taste

    Pepper, herb seasonings

    Whole-wheat bread (or pita)

    Alfalfa sprouts

Carrot sticks

Celery sticks

Skim milk or iced tea

DINNER:

Chicken breast (or turkey breast)

Brown rice

Choice of following sauces: (from prepackaged mixes or from scratch)

Curry

Tomato sauce/diced tomatoes

Herb vinaigrette

Teriyaki sauce

Salsa

Garlic and olive oil

Spinach salad with nonfat dressing (or two tablespoons of flaxseed oil with vinegar)

Mandarin orange slices

Hard-boiled egg-white slices

Red onion slices

Steamed broccoli, cauliflower, squash, spinach, kale, cabbage, green beans, etc. (choose one or two each dinner)

Fresh berries (blackberries, raspberries, blueberries, strawberries) for dessert

TABLE 9.2

HEALTHY SAMPLE DAILY MENU
(VEGETARIAN)

BREAKFAST:

Mix together:

One cup nonfat or 1-percent-fat cottage cheese

One tablespoon flaxseed oil

One cup chopped fresh fruit (berries, apples, apricots, peaches, etc.)

One glass juice (orange, grapefruit, grape, apple, etc.)

LUNCH:

Baked potato with a half cup of nonfat yogurt and chives (other low-fat baked potato condiments are: fat-free cheeses, salsa, picante sauce, barbecue sauce, low-fat salad dressings, herb seasonings)

Salad of mixed greens with low-fat dressing or vinaigrette

One raw apple

One glass of skim milk

DINNER:

One cup cold Gazpacho soup

One and one-half cups of cooked lima beans (or other type of beans or green peas)

One cup or one ear of boiled corn

One cup of mustard greens, steamed

One cup of nonfat yogurt with one-quarter cup fresh chopped walnuts (or hazelnuts or chestnuts) for dessert

One glass of skim milk

TABLE 9.3

BAD SAMPLE DAILY MENU
(WHAT YOU SHOULD NOT EAT)

BREAKFAST:

Two cups of coffee with cream and sugar

Two slices of white bread toast with a pat of margarine each

Two strips of bacon

Two eggs, sunny side up, fried in bacon drippings

One glass orange juice

LUNCH:

Ham and cheese sandwich from fast-food restaurant

Cola soft drink (and another in the afternoon)

One bag of potato chips

One pickle

DINNER:

Chicken-fried steak with gravy

One helping of mashed potatoes with margarine (made with whole milk)

One serving of green peas with a pat of margarine

One cup of whole milk

One small bowl of vanilla ice cream

TABLE 9.4

COMPARING THE DAILY MENUS

	Healthy Meat	Healthy Vegetarian	Bad Menu
Calories	1420	2000	2800
Wholeness Index	82%	108%	50%
Cholesterol (milligrams)	178	22	765
% Protein	31	24	16
% Carbohydrates	43	50	40
% Fat	26	26	44
Saturated fat (grams)	8	9	60
Polyunsaturated fat (grams)	22	26	20
Monounsaturated fat (grams)	11	23	56
Deficiencies (below RDA levels for entire day)	calcium, zinc, oopper	none	fiber, vitamin E, manganese copper, calcium magnesium, potassium

TABLE 9.5

10

Nutritional Defense against Specific Joint Problems

Your body remembers a bump on the knee, a dislocated shoulder, a sprained ankle, and other bodily insults–even though the original injury is long gone. Old injuries, however, can resurface later in the guise of osteoarthritis. Doctors call this "secondary osteoarthritis," meaning that it's caused by some former trauma to connective tissue. "Primary osteoarthritis," on the other hand, has no known cause and might be related to some existing defect in cartilage.

In both types of osteoarthritis (and as we've seen in previous chapters), there's a switch from tissue building to tissue destruction. This makes osteoarthritis a "metabolic" disorder, rather than a purely inflammatory or mechanical one. Something has gone awry in the way chondrocytes (cartilage cells) do their job. In healthy joints, cartilage is manufactured and maintained without incident. But in osteoarthritis, there's a disruption in this process– in the normal metabolism of cartilage. Cartilage starts to soften, then becomes pitted and frayed. Finally, it wears away altogether. As explained earlier, chondroprotective nutrients help restore the tissue-rebuilding process to normal.

It's important to look at the many injuries that can lead to secondary osteoarthritis, particularly in regard to what happens to joints after they've been damaged. That way, by intervening early with nutritional weapons, you can further protect yourself from later consequences.

Accidents Do Happen

■ Injuries can be either acute or chronic. A sudden blow to the joint is an example of an acute injury. There's usually a rapid change in the joint structure, including damage to cartilage. Chronic joint injuries happen over time, the result of repetitive motion or overuse. Safe, normal movements for one person might be painful and hazardous for another. Your best friend might be able to run in marathons every year, while you can barely jog a block without hurting.

Injuries are also classified as either intentional or unintentional. Being hit over the head by an intruder or assaulted by a mugger are intentional injuries. But if your knee slams into the dashboard during a car crash or you twist your ankle sliding into home plate, you've been injured unintentionally—accidentally, in other words.

Most unintentional injuries occur as a result of accidents, job-related activities, and sports injuries. Accidents are a leading cause of injuries, particularly traffic accidents, which annually cost billions to treat.

You can get hurt on the job, too. Like other injuries, occupational injuries are either acute or chronic. Having a forklift run over your foot is an example of an acute injury. Typing on a computer keyboard all day long can lead to a chronic injury such as carpal tunnel syndrome in susceptible people. During the 1990s, companies seeking to cut health-care costs have focused on "ergonomics," a method of correcting the way people perform the physical requirements of their jobs. Wearing weight belts to ease the strain of lifting and fitting computer workstations with special arm rests are examples of ergonomic efforts in the workplace.

Injuries from sports and exercise are on the rise as more people take to the track, gym, or playing field to get in shape. This shouldn't discourage you from exercising, though. Most sports injuries are mild and cause no permanent harm. In fact, 71 percent of these injuries are "minor," meaning you're out of action less than a week; 20 percent are moderate (one to three weeks lost); and only 9 percent are severe (more than three months lost). So keep your exercise program going. If you don't have one, start!

As for long-term damage with sports injuries, about 11 percent of patients still have complaints after two years, usually from sprains. About 10 percent of all sports injuries require surgery.

Sports injuries can also be acute or chronic. Many chronic injuries occur in running, one of the most unforgiving sports. About one-third of all runners report problems, probably from repetitive pounding, but only one in seven go to a doctor about it. If you're a runner, you help avoid damage to otherwise healthy joints by running on softer surfaces, wearing the proper shoes and/or adding cushioned inserts, warming up first, paying attention to pain, and sticking to a nutrient-rich diet.

Many chronic injuries are potential forerunners of osteoarthritis. Here's a look at some of the more common.

Oh, My Aching Low Back

■ Chances are, you'll have at least one bout with low-back pain in your life. In people under forty-five years old, low-back pain is the most common form of disability. The older you get, the more likely you're apt to have it. Treating low-back pain costs up to an estimated $100 billion a year.

You can get low-back pain from any number of things. Some of the more obvious sources of low-back pain are improper lifting techniques, poor back strength, and sudden movements that strain the muscles in the back. A herniated (slipped) disc in the spine also causes low-back pain, although this condition accounts for only 5 percent of all back disorders. This injury occurs when discs bulge and put pressure on nearby nerves, causing pain.

A more common cause of low-back pain, especially as you get older, is "spinal stenosis," otherwise known as degeneration of the spine. A bony overgrowth forms around vertebra, constricting the spinal-cord canal and other nerves. Symptoms include leg pain, cramps, numbness, and tingling on the thighs and calves.

Another manifestation of spinal deterioration is sciatica, in which the nerves serving the legs become pinched. This causes painful muscle spasms, stiffness upon bending over, and pain shooting into the leg from the lower back.

Other less obvious causes are smoking and riding in cars. Every time a person lights up, oxygen and circulation are decreased, hampering the supply of nutrients to tissue. One of the areas that suffers greatly is the spine. Its sheer length and intricate, sandwiched layers of ligaments and discs make it difficult for nutrients to reach every nook and cranny. So any nutritional blockade impairs the ability of discs to maintain and repair themselves.

The vibration of riding in cars jiggles and juggles nutrients away from the disc, too. If you're ever traveling long distances in a vehicle, it's a good idea to take frequent rest breaks. On your break, walk around to stimulate circulation and the diffusion of nutrients into discs.

Low-Back Pain Is Really a Nutritional Problem

■ And it's no wonder, considering the structure of the spinal column. The discs between the vertebra are doughnut-shaped pieces of cartilage. In some people, they are one-fourth to a half-inch thick. That's a long distance for microscopic nutrients such as oxygen and glucose to travel to nourish chondrocytes, the cartilage cells in the discs.

At the doughnut-hole centers of the discs is a stiff gel called the nucleus pulposus. It gets shortchanged the most, because it's the farthest removed from nutritional supplies. The nucleus is encircled by a series of tough, ring-like layers of cartilage. This structure enables the disc to withstand compression from any angle.

Without nutrients, the nucleus begins to lose the water that makes it so compliant. Over time, the nucleus starts getting harder, while the layers around it become drier and more brittle. Any wrong body movement—such as lifting a heavy object or twisting the back out of line—can force the nucleus to push its layers out farther. Or worse yet, the nucleus can shoot through its layers, like the spitting out of a watermelon seed. This is what happens with a slipped disc. Both consequences change the anatomy of the spine, pinching nerves or obstructing the movement of the vertebrae. The result is low-back pain and inflexibility.

Even under the best circumstances, nutrition to disc cells is barely sufficient for normal tissue maintenance. Any insult to the back, no matter how small, can thwart the ability of those cells to repair themselves.

Undernourished disc cells set the stage for a lot of aches and pains. Suppose you've bent over hundreds of times to pet your dog. Then one day, something in your back snaps, and you've got intense pain. The difference has to do with the nutritional health of the disc. It could no longer support that familiar movement. You injured yourself.

Although there are many causes of low-back pain, inadequate nutrition of the discs in the spinal column is at the root of the problem. If the repair mechanism of the chondrocytes in discs could somehow be stimulated, it's likely you'd feel a lot less low-back pain. But there are no drugs, physical therapies, or surgical cures that do this. All current treatments for low-back pain overlook one key fact: The metabolism of disc chondrocytes is a critical underlying factor in low-back pain.

Shouldering the Hurt

■ Swinging a tennis racquet, swimming laps, throwing a softball, and other similar repetitive motions can take their toll on the shoulder joint. One of the most common sites for injury is the rotator cuff, a part of the shoulder joint that rubs on the upper-arm bone. Untreated, the injury can progress from inflammation to degeneration of joint structures to deterioration of the entire rotator cuff.

There are different symptoms at different stages, including pain, shoulder weakness, grinding, and swelling. In the final stages, tears in the connective tissues, ruptures in the tendons of the arms, and changes in bone are frequently seen symptoms. In most cases, it takes about twenty years for the rotator cuff to fully deteriorate. Baseball fans will recognize this as a fairly common affliction among pitchers.

Not all shoulder overuse problems are sports-related. People in jobs who frequently lift loads overhead are at risk. One documented example is a fifty-three-year-old woman who worked in a cheese factory. After she had stacked more than twenty tons of cheese on shoulder-height shelves in two years, her shoulder joints had deteriorated so much that bone was rubbing against bone. She was forced to end her career and go on disability.

Elbowing Health Aside

■ Everyone is familiar with tennis elbow. You don't have to swing a racquet hitting a ball over a net to know this. However, many other repetitive arm movements can overload the tendons attached to the elbow joint. Inflammation sets in, causing pain. Playing tennis, shaking hands, opening doors, or turning a screwdriver all become painful activities. Since we always use our elbows, it's no surprise that some damage can almost always be found in elbow joints.

Knee-Deep in Pain

■ Knees are used practically nonstop. This makes them very vulnerable to injury. Young athletes who do a lot of running, jumping, or hurdling often get Jumper's Knee, an inflammation of the tendon that attaches the lower knee cap to its muscle. The damaged tendons rub on joint structures just below the knee. Bending the knees and climbing or descending stairs are painful. It usually takes several months for the knee to heal.

With the continuing boom in running and jogging, many exercisers have suffered from the ominous-sounding "iliotibial band syndrome." This affects a band of connective tissue that drapes over the bony part of your outer knee. At each foot strike, this band rubs normally over knee and thigh structures. But being bowlegged, running on sloped surfaces, or having pronated feet all cause excessive rubbing on the knee joint. Pain and inflammation set in. When you stop running, the pain stops. But "running through the pain" makes the pain so intolerable that you could be forced to stop.

Another mouthful of a knee problem is "chondromalacia patellae." This is caused by a misalignment of the kneecap. The kneecap is either structurally abnormal or has been knocked out of line by an injury. As such, the connecting muscles and tendons can't keep the kneecap in its proper groove. It hurts to sit for long stretches, although straightening the knees relieves the pain. When you're climbing stairs or getting up from a chair, your knees make quite a racket, clicking and creaking with every move. They might also lock up or suddenly buckle.

Unchecked, the surface of the kneecap, which is capped with cartilage, softens and becomes damaged. Because the knee cap moves every time you move, any abnormal force on it aggravates the damage, accelerating cartilage degeneration.

Lower Leg Injuries Leave Their Mark

■ The constant pounding of the legs on hard surfaces during running, aerobic dancing, or marching can cause a painful condition known as shin splints. The front of the calf feels tender and starts to ache. This is the result of an inflammation of the membrane covering the shin bone and/or the tendons that connect it to the front calf muscles.

Shin splints don't involve joints directly, although the pain affects how you move while exercising. A change in movement can potentially put more stress on other joints, causing them to wear more quickly.

The extreme of shin splints is the stress fracture. Continuing to run or exercise with shin splints can cause tiny microfractures in the shinbone. The bone can't adapt fast enough to the extra stress. Tendons begin to pull away from the bone, causing inflammation. Eventually, the bone/tendon connection, as well as the underlying bone, weakens. The bone can even tear apart.

At the fracture site, hardness or bumps might appear as callus formation begins. But with rest, most fractures heal within six to eight weeks. You can then resume activity at a modified pace. Like shin splints, stress fractures can have an indirect effect on joints.

Ankle and Foot Joints

■ Any repetitive stress such as running, jumping, or aerobic dancing can put cartilage-damaging impact on the joints of the ankles and feet. So can wearing shoes that fit poorly, whether or not you exercise. In fact, pushing feet into shapes that don't fit them can cause painful foot and toe deformities.

One of the foot areas most vulnerable to stress is the arch. Its stiff joints can be slowly transformed into flat feet and other abnormalities. When you walk, run, or exercise, the ankle, knee, and hip joints must then absorb more impact shock. This increases the potential for more wear-and-tear joint degeneration.

Nerves running through the foot are frequently subjected to chronic compression, causing pain, tingling, numbness, or a burning sensation in the feet and toes. Nerve damage doesn't directly affect the joints. But people who experience it often compensate for the pain by walking in such a way to avoid it. This places uneven stress on other joints and can cause joint degeneration and the eventual erosion of cartilage.

Heel problems stem from the formation of bone spurs, as well as from a condition known as plantar fascitis, in which the muscles and tendons covering the heel pad become inflamed. Sometimes, bone spurs grow into the path of the Achilles tendon, causing discomfort and even calcification (hardening) of the tendon. Heel problems can force you to change your gait, and this potentially places undue stress on joints.

Jawbone Aches and Pain

■ Joint degeneration can strike the temporomandibular joint (TMJ). Your TMJ is a hinged joint that connects your jaw to your skull. You can feel it by touching your fingers just in front of your lower ear and opening and closing your mouth.

The TMJ is different from other joints because it contains fibrocartilage, a special kind of cartilage that has a limited blood supply. A small disc of fibrocartilage in the TMJ prevents bones from rubbing against each other.

The TMJ has received a lot of attention because of a disorder called TMJ Syndrome. TMJ Syndrome is not a degenerative condition of the joint, but rather a type of pain in the muscles of the face caused by spasms of the chewing muscles. There may also be clicking or popping noises when you chew or open your mouth. Pain is usually worse in the morning—the result of clenched or grinding teeth at night. Up to 85 percent of all TMJ pain is probably muscular in origin. Severe emotional stress leads to TMJ Syndrome, and women have it more than men. All ages can get TMJ Syndrome.

Any prior trauma or rearrangement of the TMJ can lead to degenerative TMJ disease. Like osteoarthritis, symptoms appear gradually.

How do you know whether you've got TMJ Syndrome or degenerative TMJ? Unlike TMJ Syndrome, TMJ degeneration doesn't cause much pain in the morning. Instead, pain gets worse as the day goes on, and you can feel it at the joint, not in the chewing muscles.

Early and proper diagnosis is vital. There's a good chance degenerative TMJ can be healed if the disc inside the joint is undamaged. Otherwise, degeneration will continue.

HEALING THE HURTS

■ In Table 10.1 (page 158), you'll find something called a "protocol." This simply means a plan of action. It includes a list of nutrients that when used properly can benefit joint health.

You might ask: Have these protocols been scientifically validated?

No, you won't find these exact protocols tested in large scientific studies—for two reasons. First, scientists rarely do research on combinations of nutrients or drugs. When setting up studies, they're trained to narrow down test variables until only one or two remain. That's the essence of the "scientific method." Second, much of the scientific information presented here is relatively new. So there hasn't been enough time to conduct trials.

However, these protocols are based on strong scientific evidence, as presented in my previous book, *Nutrition Applied to Injury Rehabilitation and Sports Medicine.* Each nutrient listed has its own evidence. The protocols simply combine the evidence into a coherent, common-sense combination.

When your body has to fight back, whether in response to injury, illness, or everyday metabolic processes, it mobilizes a force of nutrients, all used simultaneously. These nutrients are like links in a chain. The chain is joint health. As you know, a chain is only as strong as its weakest link. No matter how indestructible the links are, one old, rusty link can break, thus rendering the entire chain useless.

This is why combinations of nutrients taken at proper doses work so effectively in real-life situations. This protocol isn't a shotgun approach, however. It's more like a coordinated missile strike, with some well-aimed smart bombs poised to hit specific targets of joint health.

Nutrients for Injuries

■ The joint injuries discussed in this section are all associated with inflammation. Most are acute injuries, although some like tendinitis can be classified as chronic. As Table 10.2 (page 161) shows, the first line of nutritional defense should be with anti-inflammatory nutrients. If a return to normal comes slowly, try the osteoarthritis protocol to accelerate the healing of your joints.

SPRAINS AND LIGAMENT TEARS

You accidentally stumble coming down your front porch steps. The weight of your body twists your foot into an unnatural position. Ouch—you've just sprained your ankle.

Sprains occur when a sudden twist or stretch forces the joint beyond its usual limits. Sprains can involve all joint structures, but especially capsules, ligaments, tendons, synovium, sheaths, and cartilage. The joint capsule and ligaments can be stretched or torn, depending upon the severity of injury. At the moment a joint is sprained, you might hear a popping or ripping sound as ligaments are torn. Pain, tenderness, swelling, bleeding under the skin, bruising, and inability to use the joint are the usual indications of a sprain.

The most commonly sprained joints are the ankles, knees, low back, neck, wrists, and fingers. Each joint follows a slightly different course of inflammation and healing. Because the cells that live in and repair ligaments are few in number, it often takes a long time for the body to repair the damage.

Ligament tears are sprains of the worst kind. Some joints, such as the knee joint, have internal and external ligaments susceptible to tearing. Frequently, more than one ligament is torn, depending upon the severity of the force involved. Contact injuries to the leg or knee area are the most common cause of ligament tears. Sometimes, noncontact ligament tears occur after pivoting or jumping awkwardly.

With ligament tears, healing is slow, often lasting months or years. Unlike bone, the repaired ligament is never as good as the original. It's about 30 to 50 percent weaker. However, chronic passive motion exercise performed by a qualified physical therapist or rehabilitation specialist can accelerate healing and return it to useful strength.

STRAINS

If you've ever pushed just a little too hard in the gym, you know what a strain is: a pulled muscle from overworking a body part. In severe strains, muscle fibers, tendon attachments, or both can actually tear.

One of the muscles most vulnerable to strains is the hamstring at the back of the thighs. This injury is the so-called charley horse.

In extreme cases of strains, tendons can be ruptured or even ripped from bones or joints. A frequently seen type of strain is the Achilles tendon rupture just above the ankle. You feel it suddenly, like something just hit or struck the back of your lower leg. Almost immediately, you're unable to stand on the ball of your foot, stand on your toes, or push off from your heels to walk. Any activity or sport requiring rapid accelerations and decelerations such as running, jumping, or playing racquet sports sets the stage for an Achilles tendon rupture.

Tendons take a long time to heal. After inflammation subsides (about four to ten days), repair begins. In about two weeks, a "tendon callus" forms. So do adhesions, which are undesirable fibers of collagen that attach to the lining of the tendon. Tendons can't move very well as a result, and function in the limb could be lost. Adhesions can contract, altering the muscular forces on joints. Muscular weakness from adhesions also changes the nature of forces on a joint. Charley horse injuries are a good example. These place abnormal strains on the kneecap, eventually producing arthritic changes in knees.

At first, tendons are slow to regain their former strength. This usually happens after remodeling, which can take as long as four to sixteen weeks. As with ligament strength, chronic passive motion exercise can speed up healing and prevent adhesions.

MENISCAL TEARS

The menisci are like little cartilage washers inside joints. In the knee joint, they separate the ends of the thigh bone and the lower leg bone. Their job is to distribute forces evenly on the cartilage in the knee, and their wedged shape helps stabilize the knee joint. The menisci also disperse synovial fluid to cartilage, aiding in joint lubrication and cartilage nutrition.

Any sudden, excessive impact can tear the meniscus. In fact, about two-thirds of all knee injuries are related to meniscal damage. Usually, injuries to other joint structures in the knee are accompanied by meniscal tears.

About six to ten hours after the tear, the knee might swell and lose flexibility. There might be some pain. Meniscal tears are usually diagnosed by X-rays or arthroscopy, a special method of viewing the inside of knee joints. If proper rest, exercise, and nutrition are followed, meniscal tears can heal on their own.

In severe cases, surgery might be required to remove the damaged portion of the meniscus. In the past, the meniscus was thought to be an expendable tissue, like the appendix, and surgeons would remove it. But then the picture changed: Various studies found that 60 percent of patients who had their knee menisci removed developed arthritic symptoms ten to fifteen years after surgery. The goal of meniscal surgery today is to leave as much of the tissue intact as possible. Even so, people with meniscal tears (treated or untreated) tend to have a higher rate of osteoarthritis.

DISLOCATIONS

This refers to a joint that is pulled out of its place. Most dislocations occur in the shoulder joint, usually after the arm is suddenly yanked or forced out of its natural position. You might feel a slipping sensation or hear a popping noise, followed by pain.

Dislocations range from mild to severe. Mild dislocations only involve injury to the joint capsule, and the bones stay in alignment. Even so, these injuries hurt and can swell. Severe dislocations break the capsule and tear ligaments. These injuries can cause arthritic changes in the affected joint later in life.

FRACTURES

These are broken bones caused by too much force hitting the bone. Bones can be fractured in many ways. A tumble down the stairs or a bruising tackle to a running back with a foot planted while making a cut are among the myriad ways one can fracture a bone. Usually, a fracture is a crack that doesn't break the bone into pieces. The crack might be tiny (called a hairline fracture), or extensive and shaped like a spiral (called a greenstick fracture). Complete breakage of the bone into adjoining pieces is called a closed compound fracture. Fractures where the broken bone protrudes from the skin are called open compound fractures. Other types of fractures include crush fractures, in which a heavy weight or force has broken the bone into small fragments, and epiphyseal fractures, caused by crushing, cracking, or breaking the growth of long bones (epiphysis) in young people.

You can also fracture bones from overuse or repetitive motion. Bone repair can't keep up with the continual and damaging stress. Take running, for example. The constant foot strike on the pavement concentrates force on your legs, causing microscopic cracks or tiny cavities in the bone. It might be a long time before you feel any pain. Extended rest from the repetitive activity usually gives the bone time to heal.

Fractures affect joint health in several ways. First, the fracture might abut the joint or even pierce it. Both can alter joint structure for the worse. Second, the fractured area might have to be immobilized, with either a cast or inactivity. Disuse can weaken and degenerate the joint. Third, a fracture might heal incorrectly, changing the angle at which the bone inserts in the joint or on how the joint accepts load forces.

BRUISES

Blows, falls, or other trauma can cause bruises. There's bleeding under the skin formed by an accumulation of blood (hematoma).

BURSITIS

This is an inflammation of the bursae, which are fluid-filled sacs that protect tendons in their movements near joints. Bursitis can occur around any joints that have bursae, including the shoulder, elbow, hip, and knee. The sacs might be injured by an acute blow or by overuse of muscles. The result is swelling and pain near the joint. If bursitis is constant, surgery can remove the offending bursal sac. However, this might create long-term problems, because bursa removal changes your joint anatomy.

There's a type of bursitis called housemaid's knee resulting from irritation and mechanical damage to the bursae around the kneecap. These sacs normally protect tendons in the knee from rubbing too much during motion. But if you're constantly kneeling or crawling on hard surfaces (such as washing a floor the old-fashioned way, on hands and knees), the bursae around the kneecap become squashed and damaged. This causes inflammation, pain, and swelling. This chronic injury is also common in contact sports such as wrestling, where the knee frequently hits the ground hard. Since the bursae are involved, knee joint structure is usually unaffected.

TENDINITIS

Any minor injury or overuse can produce tendinitis, a soreness in joints caused by a small tear or inflammation of a tendon. One of the most common sites for tendinitis is in the elbow, more commonly known as tennis elbow. You don't have to be a tennis player to get it, though. Any repetitive motion, such as raking leaves, painting a house, or pitching a baseball (Little Leaguers included) can produce tiny tears in the tendon that connects the lower arm to the elbow.

Another type of common tendinitis is Achilles tendinitis, which occurs where the Achilles tendon meets the ankle bone. Pain and swelling of the tendon sheath are the usual symptoms. Achilles tendinitis develops gradually. It doesn't directly affect the interior of joints, although it might cause other mechanical problems. These lead to degeneration of the joint.

Skin Damage

■ With many acute joint injuries comes skin damage. Or you might have skin wounds that are left over from surgery for a degenerative joint condition. In either case, supplementation might help accelerate healing.

What follows is a list of suggested supplements to try. If you're already taking some of these for a joint injury, adjust your intake of vitamin A and zinc. Or if you're following the suggested osteoarthritis or rheumatoid arthritis protocol, then add proteases, bioflavonoids, and curcumin. Remember to refer to Part Two for information on specific supplements, their absorption, and other hints for use.

Rheumatoid Arthritis

■ Relief from rheumatoid arthritis comes from paying closer attention to your diet, particularly the reduction of saturated fat. As we've seen in several of the research studies in this book, supplements have tremendous nutritional influence as well. Which is why I've included a protocol for rheumatoid arthritis, outlined in Table 10.4 (page 163). It emphasizes inflammation-fighting nutrients, as well as immune-system protectors, such as the antioxidants. Omega-3 fats are recommended, too, because several clinical trials have proved that these nutrients stimulate good prostaglandins that help reduce pain, tenderness, and stiffness.

Nutritional Protocols Made Easy

■ In following these protocols, split your total daily amounts into two or three doses taken during the day. The best times to take supplements are after breakfast, at lunch, after dinner, and before bed. Why those times? It's easier to remember at those intervals, plus taking supplements with food helps the absorption of nutrients in them.

For convenience, make up packs of supplements ahead of time by placing them in squares of aluminum foil, cupcake cups, or small plastic baggies.

As you shop around for nutritional supplements, try to match the specific nutrients listed in these protocols to product labels.

Because there are so many nutritional products on the market, you probably won't find an exact match. Just try to get close. Be sure to distinguish between mg (milligrams) and mcg (micrograms) on the labels. I've provided ranges of nutrients to make it easier for you to find products that fit these lists.

NUTRITIONAL SUPPLEMENT PROTOCOL
FOR OSTEOARTHRITIS, LOW-BACK PAIN,
AND CHRONIC JOINT INJURIES

Nutrient	Daily Amount
Glucosamine salts	1,500 mg
(Glucosamine hydrochloride (preferred), glucosamine sulfate (double dosage), N-acetylglucosamine (less than ideal))	
Chondroitin sulfates	1,500 mg
(look for purified source; avoid cartilage powders, trachea powder, mussels)	
Niacinamide (vitamin B3) (*not* niacin)	250 mg every 3-4 hours (see Table 9.1 on page 131)
Antioxidants	
Vitamin C (buffered or mineral ascorbates preferred)	1,000 to 4,000 mg
Vitamin E (d-alpha-tocopherol or mixed tocopherols; avoid dl- forms or tocopherol forms)	400 or 800 IU (mg)
Selenium (selenite or selenomethionine or both)	200 mcg
Beta Carotene	25,000 IU (15 mg)
Multiple vitamin/mineral product	Variable number, depends on content
Vitamin A (retinyl palmitate)	5,000 IU

Vitamin B1 (thiamin)	20 to 100 mg
Vitamin B2 (riboflavin)	50 mg
Vitamin B3 (niacinamide)	20 to 100 mg
Vitamin B6 (pyridoxine)	10 to 50 mg
Vitamin B12 (cyanocobalamin)	10 to 100 mcg
Folic Acid	400 mcg
Pantothenate	100 mg
Biotin (optional)	100 to 300 mcg
Vitamin C (optional)	not necessary in multi product
Vitamin D (D3 or cholecalciferol)	100 to 400 IU
Vitamin E (optional)	not necessary in multi product
Calcium (citrate, citrate-malate, lysinate)	200 to 500 mg
Magnesium (glycinate, citrate, aspartate)	200 to 500 mg
Iron	NONE, unless prescribed by doctor
Zinc (methionate, citrate, picolinate)	15 to 25 mg
Manganese (ascorbate, gluconate)	5 to 15 mg
Copper (any form)	2 to 5 mg

Chromium (polynicotinate or picolinate)	100 to 300 mcg
Selenium (optional)	100 to 300 mcg
Boron (borate)	3 to 6 mg
Iodine (optional)	50 to 150 mcg

OPTIONAL:

Bioflavonoids (citrus, silymarins, green tea, etc.)	2,000 mg

Pantothenate	2,000 mg

TIP: Other ingredients are entirely optional, but might drive cost higher.

TIP: Ask for iron-free multiple vitamin/mineral supplement.

TIP: Look first at amount of selenium and chromium on the label claim. If the amount is close to doses listed above, then the rest of the product should also fit the guidelines listed above. This is a quick way to determine the quality and completeness of a multiple vitamin/mineral product.

TIP: If you also take additional antioxidants, the amounts of vitamin C, vitamin E, and beta carotene in a multiple vitamin/mineral are not important.

TABLE 10.1

JOINT-INJURY PROTOCOL:
SPRAINS, LIGAMENT TEARS, STRAINS, MENISCAL TEARS, DISLOCATIONS, FRACTURES, BRUISES, BURSITIS, AND TENDINITIS

Nutrient	Total Daily Amount
Protease product (trypsin/chymotrypsin, bromelain, papain)	5 or 10 tablets four times daily
Vitamin C	4,000 mg
Bioflavonoids	2,000 mg
Curcumin	2,000 mg

OPTIONAL:

Multiple Vitamin/Mineral	see Osteoarthritis Protocol
Antioxidants	see Osteoarthritis Protocol
Glucosamine salts	see Osteoarthritis Protocol

TABLE 10.2

NUTRIENT SUPPLEMENTS FOR SKIN DAMAGE, SURGERY, LACERATIONS, AND ABRASIONS

Nutrient	Total Daily Amount
Protease product	see Joint Injury Protocol
Vitamin C	4,000 mg
Bioflavonoids	2,000 mg
Zinc (methionate, citrate, picolinate)	50 mg for four weeks
Vitamin A (Retinyl palmitate)	25,000 IU for two weeks
Curcumin	2,000 mg

TABLE 10.3

RHEUMATOID ARTHRITIS PROTOCOL

Nutrient	Total Daily Amounts
Multiple vitamin/mineral	same as Osteoarthritis Protocol
Antioxidants	same as Osteoarthritis Protocol
Omega-3 oils (choice of fish oils or flaxseed oil)	
Fish body oil (not fish liver oil)	9 capsules
Flaxseed oil	2 tablespoons or 6 capsules
GLA oils	6 capsules
(choice of borage, black currant seed or evening primrose oil as sources)	
Pantothenate (a B vitamin)	2,000 mg
Glucosamine salts	1,500 mg
Chondroitin Sulfates	1,500 mg

OPTIONAL:

Bioflavonoids	2,000 mg
(citrus, silymarins, Gingko biloba, green tea, etc.)	
Niacinamide	250 mg every 3 to 4 hours
(see Table 9.1 on page 131)	
Copper (Histidine salt)	10 mg copper for three months
L-Histidine (an amino acid)	10,000 mg
Curcumin	1,000 mg

TABLE 10.4

PART FOUR

Conventional Treatments: Only Part of the Answer

11

Rating the Arthritis Drugs

When you're in pain, relief is as close as the medicine cabinet—or is it?

A few years ago, while attending a regional meeting of the American Medical Association (AMA), I listened to a rheumatologist discuss drug treatments for injuries and degenerative joint disease. He talked mostly about the chemical makeup of available drugs instead of their effects. As for drug treatments, he painted a bleak picture! Although drugs reduce pain, they don't stop the progression of osteoarthritis. It just gets worse, regardless of what you take for relief, until the only solution is something drastic such as joint replacement or joint fusion. In fact, by reducing pain, more activity might actually hasten joint degeneration because the body's "wisdom" (pain) has been overridden. What's more, the side effects of some drugs are intolerable.

During the question-and-answer session, I asked him if he had heard about the new chondroprotective agents. He had, but knew no details.

That's a typical response among doctors across the U.S.—doctors want to help their patients get better, but are frustrated by conventional treatments and the lack of a real cure.

What Are Conventional Treatments?

■ Doctors have standard methods for treating acute joint injuries. If you're hurt in a car wreck, for example, there's a three-stage approach to treatment:

- ◆ First is immediate care, which gets inflammation under control so healing won't be delayed.
- ◆ The second stage concentrates on restoring joint motion and muscle strength.
- ◆ The last stage is rehabilitation; it gets you on your feet again, and back to work or in the game.

If you're a professional athlete, treatment is usually quite aggressive, since your livelihood depends on physical performance. Table 11.1 lists some of the more common treatments for sports or joint injuries.

With osteoarthritis and other degenerative joint diseases, your doctor might recommend some "general treatments." Given to everyone with joint diseases at one time or another, these general treatments include weight reduction, an exercise program suited to your fitness level and conditioning, and pain-reducing drugs.

Drugs represent one of the conventional ways to treat joint diseases. There are many different types of drugs for osteoarthritis, ranging from over-the-counter medications to powerful prescription drugs.

But are arthritis drugs the best medicine? Are they hurting or helping treatment? What works and what doesn't? Let's look at how the major arthritis medications stack up:

Aspirin: A Mixed Blessing

■ Aspirin (technically acetylsalicylic acid) is the most widely available and inexpensive of the class of drugs known as nonsteroidal anti-inflammatory drugs (NSAIDs). Aspirin is the drug of first choice for relieving pain in rheumatoid arthritis, although that's no longer the case with osteoarthritis. It comes plain, buffered, coated, timed-released, effervescent, or paired with other compounds such as acetaminophen or sodium bicarbonate. Other types of salicylates are also available. Researchers frequently use aspirin as the yardstick to measure newer-generation arthritis drugs in clinical trials.

> *Aspirin is like a hit man hired to kill the bad guys.*

You take aspirin to ease the pain or to control inflammation. For pain, the typical dosage is up to about two thousand milligrams; for inflammation, some people are required to take up to four thousand milligrams daily.

One brand of aspirin calls it "the wonder drug that works wonders." But how does aspirin actually work?

Aspirin kills off an enzyme that makes prostaglandins, known scientifically as eicosanoids (eye-COE-sah-noids). Made from fat, prostaglandins are either good or bad, as explained earlier. The good ones reduce pain and inflammation; the bad ones produce them. When cells are damaged, they release prostaglandins. If you have osteoarthritis, your cells, including those around and in joints, make more of the bad kind.

Aspirin is like a hit man hired to kill the bad guys. But the problem is, aspirin can't tell the bad guys from the good. So a lot of innocent bystanders (the good prostaglandins) get knocked off in the hit. That's why aspirin has some pretty severe side effects.

Side effects? Aspirin? No way! Hasn't aspirin been recently touted as a lifesaver in some life-threatening diseases?

While an aspirin a day may keep the cardiologist away, it's the most toxic drug you can take for osteoarthritis. The high doses often required can make you feel queasy, as well as give you a stomachache.

A more severe side effect is stomach ulcers. One reason you need good prostaglandins is to manufacture the mucus that coats the stomach lining. But aspirin kills off the prostaglandins that do this. Without any protective mucus, stomach acid and bile leak in, eroding the lining of the stomach. The result is an ulcer. There's bleeding, and the blood often shows up in stool tests for colon cancer. This gives a false reading or can mask a positive result.

At worst, aspirin can lead to a perforated stomach ulcer, in which the stomach lining is pierced. This can be deadly. In fact, due to aspirin-induced perforated ulcers, the death rate of people with osteoarthritis is 11 percent higher than for people without it. Another potentially fatal side effect of aspirin is kidney damage. And in susceptible people, aspirin is likely to produce a lethal allergic reaction. Because of these severe, potentially fatal side effects, aspirin has fallen out of favor among doctors for treating osteoarthritis.

Acetaminophen: Aspirin's Chief Rival

■ Acetaminophen rivals aspirin as a pain-stopper. But it doesn't do a good job as an anti-inflammatory. Where safety is concerned though, it beats aspirin hands down. There's no risk of bleeding ulcers because acetaminophen works differently than aspirin does. Acetaminophen might cause skin rashes, however, and overdoses can destroy the liver.

The usual daily doses are 325 to 650 milligrams taken three times a day. Doctors often recommend that elderly patients take acetaminophen at bedtime to (1) prevent disorientation from sleeping pills, and (2) relieve pain for a good night's sleep.

Narcotic Painkillers

■ When the pain is intolerable and hard to control, doctors might prescribe codeine or propoxyphene. Both are mild narcotics, which, like their stronger relatives heroine and morphine, can become addicting.

With either drug, you might have to contend with dizziness, disorientation, drowsiness, nausea, or vomiting. Doctors usually use these drugs against pain flare-ups on a temporary basis only.

Combination products such as Tylenol with Codeine seem to reduce pain better than either drug alone. Also, nonaspirin pain relievers have fewer side effects than aspirin and can be combined with other NSAIDs.

Newer Anti-Inflammatory NSAIDs

■ These NSAIDs are a group of prescription and over-the-counter drugs that have been hailed as safer alternatives to aspirin. They include Advil and Motrin (ibuprofen), Naprosyn (naproxen), and Feldene (piroxicam), among others. They're all effective pain reducers and inflammation fighters. For relief, you generally take them just twice a day. That way, it's easier to stick to your medication schedule.

These drugs tend to build up in the body, causing potentially severe side effects. A drug called benoxaprofen was removed from the market because it was associated with some deaths related to liver and kidney problems in the elderly. Butazolidin (phenylbutazone) isn't used for osteoarthritis any more because a few elderly women died of bone-marrow failure after taking it.

Like aspirin, these newer NSAIDs block the formation of prostaglandins—both the good ones and the bad. This is why NSAIDs can be toxic. Popping some ibuprofen for an occasional headache doesn't put you at risk, however. It's only at high doses that there's the potential for trouble. Osteoarthritis sufferers tend to start taking more and more pain relievers as joint damage progresses and the pain gets worse. Years of use can lead to disturbing side effects. You have to be on the lookout for these and report them immediately to your doctor. What's more, it's difficult to predict who will have a bad reaction to these drugs. Everyone is different, with a different threshold of safety.

> *Years of use can lead to disturbing side effects.*

The Dark Side of NSAIDs

■ The NSAIDs share similar side effects, with the potential to damage cartilage, the stomach, liver, kidney, immune system, skin, bone marrow, and nervous system. Perhaps the most troublesome of these for people with joint problems is the drugs' effects on cartilage.

Some NSAIDs, particularly aspirin, can actually destroy cartilage and block its repair. Numerous studies for the past twenty-five years have proved this.

When investigators added aspirin to normal and osteoarthritic cartilage cultures from animals and humans, they found that the synthesis of proteoglycans in cartilage slows down significantly. The doses used in these lab-dish cultures equaled the usual doses taken by arthritis sufferers for pain. This means that aspirin prevents cartilage from repairing itself—and speeds up the progression of osteoarthritis! In similar experiments with animal cultures, other NSAIDs inhibited cartilage synthesis, too. These include:

- ◆ diclofenac (Voltaren)
- ◆ diflunisal (Dolobid)
- ◆ fenoprofen (Nalfon)
- ◆ ibuprofen (Advil, Motrin)
- ◆ indomethacin (Indocin)
- ◆ isoxicam
- ◆ naproxen (Naprosyn, Anaprox, Aleve)
- ◆ oxyphenbutazone
- ◆ phenylbutazone (Butazolidin)
- ◆ piroxicam (Feldene)
- ◆ tolmetin (Tolectin)

Some researchers have even injected NSAIDs directly into animal joints, only to find that the drugs produced osteoarthritic changes. It has also been discovered that certain NSAIDs prevent the manufacture of collagen in joints. In an ironic twist of medical fate, the only NSAID that stimulates proteoglycans is benoxaprofen, now banned for causing liver and kidney-damage-related deaths.

A few studies have looked at what aspirin, ibuprofen, indomethacin, and naproxen do to the proteoglycan-making process in human osteoarthritic cartilage. It's not good. In osteoarthritic animals, cartilage deterioration got worse when they were fed NSAIDs in usual therapeutic doses.

Taking certain NSAIDs for osteoarthritis of the hip accelerates the breakdown of cartilage. In a 1977 study, people who took indomethacin to relieve their hip pain had further unexpected deterioration of the joint. This led researchers to coin a new term—indomethacin hips—which describes the worsening of osteoarthritis in people on this NSAID.

In another study, a group of patients (105 in all) with osteoarthritis of the hip were given either indomethacin or azapropazone (a painkiller that doesn't affect cartilage in lab-dish cultures). All the patients were awaiting total hip replacements.

Compared to the painkiller group, the indomethacin patients showed greater and more rapid deterioration of the hip. Not only that, they had to have their surgeries much sooner (by 50 percent) than the other group.

Why the rapid acceleration? One possible explanation has to do with the pain-stopping benefits of NSAIDs. When you're in less pain, you tend to move around more. Since your joints are structurally in bad shape already, any movement further hurts the cartilage. NSAIDs thus have an indirect effect on joint health. But the aforementioned study also used a non-NSAID painkiller and did not find more rapid deterioration. Combined with strong biochemical evidence that NSAIDs break down cartilage in cultures, these results mean some NSAIDs have a direct, toxic effect on cartilage.

Millions of people are taking NSAIDs for joint problems, yet most of these drugs are doing more harm than good. In light of this, it's hard to figure out why so little research has been done on humans.

To help you choose the safest and most effective pain relief for your joint problems, I've categorized the NSAIDs as either "routinely bad" or "indifferent" (see Table 11.2). In truth, none of the NSAIDs are actually good for cartilage. Because there aren't yet enough real-life experiments in humans, these assessments could change over time. But if I absolutely had to take an NSAID for osteoarthritis, I'd opt for one on the indifferent list.

From Stomachaches to Ulcers

■ Gastrointestinal side effects range from mild (diarrhea and constipation) to severe (potentially fatal ulcers). As mentioned earlier, NSAIDs *stop* production of the good prostaglandins needed to protect the stomach lining. If enough of these chemical good guys are killed off, the stomach lining can't repair itself fast enough. That puts you at risk of ulceration. An ulcer that grows can actually poke a hole in the stomach, producing what is otherwise known as a perforated ulcer. Worse yet, the ulcer might happen to erode a big blood vessel, causing internal bleeding (hemorrhaging) that's as dangerous as getting a gunshot in the stomach.

The gastrointestinal problems associated with NSAIDs are alarming. For example:

♦ Each year, painful stomach ulcers, hemorrhage, and perforated ulcers strike 2 to 4 percent of all patients taking NSAIDs.

♦ Nearly one out of every three people, or 31 percent, taking NSAIDs experienced stomach ulcers or gastritis (erosion of the stomach lining). These findings were revealed by endoscopy, a method of viewing the stomach by inserting a special tube down the throat.

♦ There are no warning signs of NSAIDs' toxicity—until it's almost too late. In more than half (58.2 percent) of people taking NSAIDs, a life-threatening incident such as massive bleeding or a perforated ulcer is the first alert of toxicity.

♦ If you're taking an NSAID for arthritis, you're six and a half times more likely to be hospitalized for stomach problems. Other factors increase your risk for side effects, too: being older than age sixty, taking corticosteroids, smoking, having a history of stomach pains, taking antacids or anti-ulcer drugs, being a diabetic, and suffering from kidney or liver disease. Incidentally, anti-ulcer drugs and antacids are only partially effective against NSAID-induced stomach ulcers.

◆ When it comes to stomach problems, the three most troublesome NSAIDs are aspirin, phenylbutazone, and indomethacin. Taking more than one NSAID at the same time can double the risk of stomach ailments.

◆ Injections of a good prostaglandin called misoprostol prevent stomach damage from NSAIDs.

The Potential for Liver Damage

■ The liver is an amazing, although underrated chemical factory in the body. It is responsible for processing all the absorbed nutrients of digestion and oxygen. It's well known that NSAIDs are toxic to the liver. When taking NSAIDs for degenerative joint disease, you should undergo regular blood tests to see how well your liver is holding up. If the tests reveal mild to moderate elevations in liver enzymes, you might have some liver damage.

Jaundice, as shown in the yellowing of the whites of your eyes, is another sign of potential trouble. But once you're off the drugs, the damage reverses itself, thanks to the liver's enormous powers of regeneration.

Chaos for Kidneys

■ With their intricate system of tubes, capillaries, and blood vessels, the kidneys are small chemical-filtration plants, regulating the composition of body fluids and producing urine. In susceptible people, NSAIDs can create havoc in this operation. Those at greatest risk include the elderly, people with pre-existing kidney disease, those on blood-pressure medication, patients with congestive heart failure or liver disease, or salt-depleted people.

Kidney problems are the second most common side effect from NSAIDs. Routine monitoring through blood tests can pick up any signs of possible damage. Sudden puffiness or water retention are symptoms, too.

Of all NSAIDs, the drug sulindac was once thought to be the least toxic to kidneys, but now it's been linked to kidney and gallbladder stones. There appears to be no NSAID that's completely safe for the kidneys.

A Chink in the Immune System Armor

■ It's possible to have a bad allergic reaction to NSAIDs, although these are rare and infrequent. If you have nasal polyps, asthmas, or sinus problems, stay away from aspirin or NSAIDs. They might induce asthma or block air passages, making it hard to breathe. Anyone with a history of itchy skin is at a higher risk of allergies to NSAIDs.

Anyone with a history of itchy skin is at a higher risk of allergies to NSAIDs.

Tolmetin and zomepirac have been known to cause potentially severe allergic reactions. For this reason, zomepirac was taken off the market in 1983. With any NSAID, it's difficult for doctors to predict who's going to have allergic reactions.

A Rash of Skin Side Effects

■ Rashes from aspirin and/or NSAIDs show up in about 3 percent of all people taking these drugs. Other reported skin problems include itching, acne, and sensitivity to sunlight. Among NSAIDs, phenylbutazone and oxyphenbutazone cause the

severest skin reactions, while piroxicam, sulindac, and meclofenamate cause the highest number of reactions.

Bone-Marrow Mayhem

■ In rare cases, NSAIDs have halted the production of blood
cells by the bone marrow, leading to an often fatal condition
called aplastic anemia, whereby red blood cells, white blood cells,
and platelets disappear and are not replaced.

Two out of every one hundred thousand people taking
phenylbutazone are victims of aplastic anemia. Other NSAIDs
(ibuprofen, piroxicam, indomethacin, sulindac, and tolmetin),
however, have very rarely caused aplastic anemia.

All NSAIDs, particularly aspirin, block the ability of platelets
to clot, causing the blood to thin. This blood thinning is reversible
when NSAIDs (except for aspirin) are stopped. People taking anticoagulant drugs or who have blood-clotting problems should
definitely consult their doctor before taking any NSAID.

Short-Circuiting the Nervous System

■ The nervous system is the communication network for the
human body, taking information from the outer world and re-
laying it to the inner world of organs, tissues, and cells. Large
doses of NSAIDs disrupt activities in the brain and spinal cord,
which together make up the message-conducting central nervous
system. High-dose aspirin takers, for example, have experienced
ringing in the ears, and hearing loss. Aspirin overdoses cause
mental confusion, hallucinations, hyperactivity, speech problems, and seizures. Coma and death have been reported as well.
If a doctor suspects an aspirin overdose, testing blood levels can
confirm it.

Likewise, other NSAIDs are known to cause memory loss, confusion, loss of concentration, loss of mental functions, changes in mood and personality, sleeplessness, depression, and even paranoia, particularly in the elderly. Some of these symptoms are chalked up to old age. This masks their true identity as drug side effects, so there's no way of telling how many people are being sidelined mentally by NSAIDs. People with lupus and other autoimmune diseases seem to be at greater risk of developing nervous system side effects from NSAIDs. If people were aware of the possibility of nervous system side effects from NSAIDs, then they would be the most reported NSAID side effects.

MUSCLE RELAXANTS

■ These are used to treat painful muscle spasms associated with injury of muscles, bones, and joints. Muscle relaxants are frequently prescribed for osteoarthritis of the spine, which is responsible for many back problems.

Colchicine: A Last Resort

■ If you have severe osteoarthritis of the spine, your doctor might prescribe colchicine, but only as a last resort. Why it helps spinal osteoarthritis is unclear, since osteoarthritis in other joints doesn't respond to colchicine. More often, colchicine is used to treat gout, a disease that produces pain and swelling around the joints, along with fever and chills. Colchicine has some serious side effects, including abdominal pain, lethal allergic reactions, and anemia. Its use must be carefully considered and monitored.

Injectable Corticosteroids

■ Corticosteroids (or steroids) are natural or synthetic reproductions of the hormones manufactured by the adrenal glands in response to stress. They control many functions in the body, from metabolism to immune response.

Few drugs can touch the inflammation-fighting power of corticosteroids. In osteoarthritis, they're sometimes used as an immediate yet temporary remedy for pain, stiffness, swelling, and inflammation. A handful of doctors inject them directly into joints. More typically, corticosteroids are injected around joints to relieve symptoms of bursitis and other joint conditions. In most cases, they're used to treat rheumatoid arthritis where there is definite inflammation going on. Even so, the benefits don't outweigh the risks for long-term use. There are some physical prices to pay.

When injected into joints multiple times over a certain period, corticosteroids actually caused osteoarthritis in animals. Early studies in humans from the fifties discovered that corticosteroids influenced the development of osteoarthritis in joints that were injected multiple times. What's more, adding these steroids to cartilage cultures promotes rapid cell damage and cartilage destruction.

Corticosteroids can damage tendons, lead to joint damage, suppress adrenal functions, degrade cartilage, and cause osteoporosis, among other suspected side effects. In most therapies for arthritis, these drugs complement conventional treatments or are used as a last-ditch effort. Doctors and researchers continue to explore ways to use corticosteroids effectively, but without the risk of long-term joint damage.

Injectable Anesthetics: Dulling the Pain

■ If you're undergoing physical therapy for a joint problem, your doctor might inject an anesthetic (usually 1-percent lidocaine) into or around certain joints. The purpose of the injection is to ease the pain. That way, you can move around better during therapy and ultimately improve your joint mobility.

The shoulder and spine are the joints most commonly injected. Usually infrequent, these injections don't cause the same long-term damage associated with corticosteroid injections.

Toward the Future

■ The drugs you're taking today are meant to relieve your pain and help you move around better. Hopefully, you'll be able to one day take a medication that stops the breakdown of cartilage without any unpleasant side effects. Until then, you have chondroprotective nutrients to do the work that drugs can't.

TREATING SPORTS INJURIES

RICE (Rest, Ice, Compression, Elevation)

....

PRINCER (Prevention, Rest, Ice, NSAIDs, Compression, Elevation, Rehabilitation)

....

Cryotherapy (cold)

....

Thermotherapy (heat) (whirlpools, paraffin baths, fluidotherapy, hydrocollator packs, diathermy, ultrasound)

....

Electrical Stimulation (TENS, EGS, interferential)

....

Massage

....

Manual Therapy

....

Traction

....

Acupuncture

....

TABLE 11.1

RATING THE NSAIDs FOR THEIR EFFECT ON CARTILAGE

Routinely Bad	Indifferent (Not Bad)
Aspirin (acetylsalicylic acid)	Acetaminophen
Other salicylates	Diclofenac
Fenoprofen	Fenbufen
Ibuprofen	Ketoprofen
Indomethacin	Piroxicam
Isoxicam	Sulindac
Naproxen	Tiaprofenic acid
Oxyphenbutazone	
Phenylbutazone	
Tolmetin	

NOTE: A rating of "Routinely Bad" means that the drug inhibited manufacture of cartilage components or led to cartilage damage in animals. An "Indifferent" rating means that the drug did not hurt cartilage.

TABLE 11.2

Sources (Table 11.2):

Arsenis, C., and J. McDonnell. "Effects of Antirheumatic Drugs on the Interleukin-1 Alpha Induced Synthesis and Activation of Proteinases in Articular Cartilage Explants in Culture." *Agents-Actions.* Supplement 27 (1989):261-264.

Bjelle, A., and I. Eronen. "The In Vitro Effect of Six NSAIDs on the Glycosaminoglycan Metabolism of Rabbit Chondrocytes." *Clin. Exp. Rheumatol.* 9 (1991):369-374.

Brandt, K. "Drug-Induced Changes in Cartilage. Do NSAIDs Influence the Outcome of Degenerative Joint Disease?" *Degenerative Joints,* Vol. 2, ed. G. Verbruggen, E. M. Veys. Amsterdam: Excerpta Medica 2 (1985) 315-323.

Brandt, K. D. "Nonsteroidal Anti-inflammatory Drugs and Articular Cartilage." *J. Rheumatol* Supplement 14 (1987):132-133.

Brandt, K. D., and D. Flusser. "Osteoarthritis," chapter 2 in *Prognosis in the Rheumatic Diseases.* ed. N. Bellamy. Dordrecht: Kluwer Academic Publishers, 1991. 11-36.

David, M. J., E. Vignon, M. J. Peschard, P. Broquet, P. Louisot, and M. Richard. "Effect of Nonsteroidal Anti-inflammatory Drugs (NSAIDS) on Glycosyltransferase Activity from Human Osteoarthritic Cartilage." *Br. J. Rheumatol.* 1992. 31 (Supplement 1):13-17.

de Vries, B. J., P. M. van der Kraan, and W. B. van den Berg. "Decrease of Inorganic Blood Sulfate Following Treatment with Selected Antirheumatic Drugs: Potential Consequences for Articular Cartilage." *Agents-Actions* 29 (1990): 224-231.

Dingle, J. T. "Prostaglandins in Human Cartilage Metabolism." *J. Lipid Mediat.* 6 (1993):303-312.

Herman, J. H., A. M. Appel, R. C. Khosla, and E. V. Hess. "The *In Vitro* Effect of Select Classes of Nonsteroidal Anti-inflammatory Drugs on Normal Cartilage Metabolism." *J. Rheumatol.* 13 (1986):1014-1018.

Kalbhen, D. A. "Degenerative Joint Disease Following Chondrocyte Injury–Chemically Induced Osteoarthritis." *Degenerative Joints*, Vol. 2. Ed. G. Verbruggen, E. M. Veys. Amsterdam: Excerpta Medica, 1985. 299-313.

Kalbhen, D. A. "The Influence of NSAIDs on Morphology of Articular Cartilage." *Scand. J. Rheumatol.* Supplement 77 (1988):13-22.

Newman, N. M., and R. S. M. Ling. "Acetabular Bone Destruction Related to Nonsteroidal Anti-inflammatory Drugs." *Lancet.* 2 (1985):11-14.

Obeid, G., X. Zhang, and X. Wang. "Effect of Ibuprofen on the Healing and Remodeling of Bone and Articular Cartilage in the Rabbit Temporomandibular Joint." *J. Oral Maxillofac. Surg.* 50 (1992):843-849.

Pelletier, J. P., J. M. Cliutier, and J. Martel-Pelletier. "*In Vitro* Effects of Tiaprofenic Acid, Sodium Salicylate and Hydrocortisone on the Proteoglycan Metabolism of Human Osteoarthritic Cartilage." *J. Rheumatol.* 16 (1989):646-655.

Rashad, S., P. Revell, A. Hemingway, F. Low, K. Rainsford, and F. Walker. "Effect of Nonsteroidal Anti-inflammatory Drugs on the Course of Osteoarthritis." *Lancet.* 2 (1989):519-522.

Ronningen, H. and N. Langeland. "Indomethacin Hips." *Acta Orthop. Scand.* 48 (1977): 556.

POSSIBLE ADVERSE SIDE EFFECTS OF NSAIDs*

Musculoskeletal
Suppression of cartilage repair and synthesis

Gastrointestinal
Stomach ulcers
Stomach perforation
Gastrointestinal bleeding
Nausea
Vomiting
Abdominal pain
Diarrhea
Constipation

Kidneys
Fluid retention
Kidney damage

Liver
Jaundice
Elevated liver enzymes in blood (nonspecific liver damage)
Liver failure

Immune system
Allergic reactions
Asthma-like symptoms (closing of airways)

Skin
Acne
Rashes
Itching
Sensitivity to sunlight
Skin eruptions

Bone marrow

Bone marrow failure (aplastic anemia)

Blood thinning (less ability to clot)

Nervous system

Ringing in ears; hearing loss

Changes in mood or personality

Confusion, memory loss, inability to concentrate

Headaches

Dizziness, lightheadedness

Drowsiness

Depression, paranoia

*NSAIDs stands for Nonsteroidal Anti-Inflammatory Drugs (listed in Table 11.4 on the following page).

TABLE 11.3

NSAIDs USED FOR JOINT PROBLEMS

Generic Name Trade Name *Comments*	Usual Daily Dosage (mg)
Aspirin Bayer, Bufferin, Anacin, many more *Most toxic NSAID, not generally recommended anymore for OA*	1,000-3,600
Acetaminophen (Paracetamol) Tylenol, many others *Pain relief only, not anti-inflammatory*	1,000-2,500
Ibuprofen Advil, Nuprin, Motrin generics *Most commonly used NSAID for joint problems; available over-the-counter or prescription*	600-2,400
Naproxen Naprosyn *Take twice daily*	500-1,000
Fenoprofen Nalfon Watch for kidney damage	800-2,400
Ketoprofen Orudis	150-300
Flurbiprofen Ansaid	200-300
Etodolac Lodine *Less stomach bleeding than other NSAIDs*	600-1,200

Phenylbutazone   100-400
  Butazolidin
  Not used much anymore; too toxic

Indomethacin   75-200
  Indocin
  Use declining because of toxicity

Sulindac   300-400
  Clinoril
  Twice daily dosing

Tolmetin   600-1,600
  Tolectin
  Watch for allergic reactions

Diclofenac   100-150
  Voltaren
  Watch for liver damage

Meclofenamate   200-400
  Meclomen
  Watch for laxative effects

Piroxicam   10-20
  Feldene
  Once daily dosing; pay close attention to kidney status

Diflunisal   500-1,000
  Dolobid
  Safer type of aspirin

Salicylic salicylate   975-3,600
  Salsalate
  Safer type of aspirin

Magnesium salicylate   1,000-3,600

Doan's Pills, Trilisate, many others

"Natural" form of aspirin, safer than aspirin, but less anti-inflammatory

TABLE 11.4

12

~

Going under the Knife: A Realistic Option?

If you're like most people, the thought of surgery strikes fear in your heart. In addition to drug therapy, surgery is one of the conventional treatments used in osteoarthritis and other degenerative joint diseases. Surgery uses invasive procedures–those that break the skin–to correct, remove, or repair bodily structures. These procedures usually entail opening the skin to gain access to parts of the body.

It used to be that many joint surgeries required large incisions, extended hospital stays, and a long, painful period of rehabilitation. Although some surgeries are still major, newer, less-invasive techniques are used to correct disabling joint problems.

The goal of surgery is to help manage the course of joint degeneration after other treatment options have failed. Most surgeries are carefully considered before being performed, since the changes in body structures are permanent. In some surgeries, there's little chance of returning to full function.

Is surgery a realistic option? For perspective on the role of surgery, here's a rundown on the various types of surgeries used to treat and manage joint disease.

Arthroscopy: Looking into Joint Disease

■ In the early seventies, a special procedure called arthroscopy was introduced for the diagnosis and treatment of joint problems. In this procedure, the arthroscopic surgeon makes a small incision on one side of the joint and inserts a tiny tube. Utilizing a special optical system, he can then view the inside of the joint on a screen or through an eyepiece. Loose pieces of cartilage, mineral deposits, meniscus, bone, synovium, joint fluid, bone spurs, and osteophytes can be removed. Clearing out the joint cavity restores the integrity of the joint. Arthroscopy works best in the earliest stages of osteoarthritis.

Compared to other surgical techniques, arthroscopy is easier on patients. There's less time to heal since the incision is so small, and you can be back on your feet in a matter of days.

Follow-up research has found that about half of all patients who undergo arthroscopy have few, if any, problems several years after their surgery. The others have temporary relief, lasting up to two years, or no relief at all.

Synovectomy: Some Success in Arthritis

■ Removing all or part of the joint lining (the synovium) is known as a synovectomy. The synovium gets inflamed in rheumatoid arthritis, so the procedure is often an option for people with this form of arthritis. Synovectomies have been tried with some success in osteoarthritis, particularly in those cases where the synovium has expanded or thickened and is blocking other joint structures. If it gets into the wrong part of the joint, the synovium can be pinched.

Tenotomy for Painful Contractures

■ Severe joint disorders often cause "contractures," in which the joint is forced into a crippling or useless angle. The hand might ball into a fist or the feet may turn inward. Contractures compromise movement and can be painful.

An operation called a tenotomy corrects contractures. In surgery, tendons are cut, relieving the muscular and mechanical stress on the affected joint. The downside of the surgery is that your joint function can be lost permanently. Even so, you'll feel better than you did before the surgery. Tenotomies are usually performed on hip joints.

Osteotomy: Realigning the Joints

■ The angle at which a bone enters its joint can be pushed way out of line by an injury, degenerative joint disease, or genetic factors. The misalignment places uneven stress on the joint, leading to cartilage damage and ultimately to osteoarthritis.

Osteotomy (oh-stee-AH-toe-me) is the surgical removal of a piece of bone to change the stress on a joint. In this procedure, the surgeon takes out a wedge-shaped or triangular piece of bone from the long bone that connects to the affected joint. As in fracture repair, the ends of the bone are kept together until they're healed. Once healed, the bone inserts into the joint at the proper angle, greatly improving joint mechanics.

Often, osteotomy stops the progression of osteoarthritis entirely; other times, it doesn't. The procedure, however, has such a high success rate that it's considered an effective surgical option for those with severe osteoarthritis. In studies, the effectiveness of osteoarthritis treatments is judged on whether patients require osteotomy operations. Fewer osteotomies are a measure of success.

Who responds best to osteotomy? People with severe osteo-arthritis in their fingers, knee, and hip joint are likely candidates. Performed on fingers, osteotomy helps prevent crippling curling of the joints. In the knee, joints are realigned by cutting and reattaching the thigh bone above the knee joint or the bones of the lower leg. Hip joints can be repositioned by cutting and refitting the thigh bone behind the hip joint or farther down. Sometimes, surgeons remove pieces of vertebra from the spine to ease the pressure on the nerves and spinal cord, but this procedure is not strictly an osteotomy.

Resection: Removing Bony Lumps

■ The bony lumps that develop in the big toe, thumb, and fingers (Heberden's nodes) are best corrected by surgical removal or "resection." As part of surgery, the surgeon can realign the joint to prevent further problems. Because it cleans out the joint, resection is similar to arthroscopy but is more invasive.

Implants: New Parts for Used Ones

■ Some joints lose their cartilage relatively quickly. Surgically, a simple, tried-and-true solution is to lay down a new surface over the joint, like a washer in a faucet. Materials range from your own soft tissue (connective tissue and fat) to silicone rubber implants. Unfortunately, the long-term success of implants hasn't been very good, so their use is dwindling. Nowadays surgeons look at joint implants as a temporary solution until other more permanent options can be pursued.

Implants are typically used in the finger, hand, wrist, and elbow joints—but not on weight-bearing joints. The forces on weight-bearing joints would literally chew up implants in no time at all. Even in non-weight-bearing joints, implants tend to degrade in months, sometimes weeks. What's worse, silicone rubber implants have been linked to inflammatory joint changes. These problems might be similar to the immune system problems seen in women with silicone breast implants.

Arthroplasty: Replacing Your Movable Parts

■ If you're crippled by advanced osteoarthritis or rheumatoid arthritis, you might want to explore a surgical procedure called arthroplasty. This is the actual replacement of joint structures with plastic, steel, or other high-tech materials. The hip, knee, elbow, shoulder, and ankle are the most commonly replaced joints. Thanks to advancements in bioengineering, this procedure is a viable treatment option for degenerative joint disease.

Depending on the joint in question, arthroplasty may be partial, one-sided, or total. Some procedures smooth the surface of only one side of the joint. In a total joint replacement, the surgeon removes both ends of the bones that make up a joint and attaches the new artificial joint connections to the remaining bone. Other joint structures, such as the synovium, tendons, ligaments, and capsules, are removed or reattached. Care is taken not to damage nearby nerves, blood vessels, and lymphatics. To prevent complications, you're given antibiotics and anticoagulants (blood thinners).

Arthroplasty has the potential to cause infection deep in the bone or joint. This can lead to infectious arthritis and necessitate the removal of the new joint. About half of all joint replacements come loose from their bone attachments in much the same way a tire separates from its axle. Fortunately, newer materials have cut this failure rate dramatically.

Arthroplasty is a major operation—and very expensive. Recovery takes a long time. There's extensive damage to soft tissue. Extended rehabilitation is needed to get you back on your feet again. The trauma of the operation means a lot of people can't safely undergo it and are eliminated from consideration. If you're a candidate for arthroplasty, pay close attention to your nutrition before and after the surgery. Good nutrition helps you recover better. Although traumatic, arthroplasty has a high, long-term success rate, providing years of pain-free or pain-reduced joint motion.

Arthrodesis: Fusing the Joints

■ When all other treatment options have failed, a last resort for joint problems is arthrodesis—removing the joint entirely and not replacing it. Though drastic and unwanted, arthrodesis for some is still better than living with constant joint pain and deterioration.

In this procedure, both ends of a joint are removed or re-shaped. All the cartilage, along with some joint structures, is taken out, too. The bone ends are fused together and allowed to heal into a single bone. Fused joints can't move. But since there's no joint, there's no longer any joint disease.

Any joint can be fused into a single joint. Arthrodesis, however, is usually performed on the vertebra of the spine, fingers, thumbs, wrists, feet, ankles, knees, and hips.

An Option to Consider

■ As conventional treatments go, surgery remains an important option, particularly since it can correct advanced stages of joint degeneration. The surgical technology now available does things once thought impossible years ago. The decision to undergo surgery must be considered with your physician. Carefully weigh all the risks against the prospect for a better quality of life.

13

Other Arthritis-Care Programs: How Well Do They Work?

Right now, your doctor is probably telling you that the only thing that can be done for your torment is to relieve the pain, primarily with drugs. You know there's no cure for the agony. But there are other treatments, some with medical backing, some without. Here's a look at several of these therapies, both conventional and not-so-conventional.

Physical Therapy: Moving Away from the Pain

■ Ever let your car sit idle in a cold garage for a long time? If you do, you must know how much trouble it is to start it up again. Your joints are the same way. Left unused, they have less get-up-and-go.

If you have arthritis, you must exercise your joints to ensure joint mobility and flexibility. One way to accomplish this is through a supervised physical therapy program—another conventional treatment for osteoarthritis and degenerative joint disease.

Certain types of therapeutic exercises will loosen your joints and help restore movement. One of the more common is passive resistance exercise. This involves range-of-motion exercises in which the physical therapist gently guides your limbs through repetitive movements. These help stimulate circulation, improve flexibility, prevent contractures, and keep the muscles in good condition. There's no forcing or stretching.

Another much-used therapeutic exercise is water exercise. Moving around in water helps you regain joint mobility and build endurance.

There's more to physical therapy than therapeutic exercise, however. Certain techniques borrowed from rehabilitation medicine have proved very valuable in treating arthritis sufferers. Manipulation, massage, and electrical stimulation are used to promote movement, relieve pain, and trigger sensation. Hot and cold therapies can help short-circuit pain. Devices like traction and splints help relieve painful contractures.

Physical therapy continues to be a vital mainstay of a comprehensive arthritis-care program. Its goal is to get you moving again. Consult your physician to find or set up an individualized program that will help you better manage your condition.

Change Your Environment

■ Perhaps your fingers are so swollen and stiff that you dial a wrong number every time you make a phone call. That can get tiresome, sometimes downright embarrassing. Or you risk a slip in the tub whenever you try to take a bath. Trying to dress in the mornings is such a chore that you'd rather stay in your robe all day. The easiest things to do have become the hardest, and sometimes the riskiest.

Some good news: There are countless products available out there—technically known as "adaptive devices"—all designed to make life easier for you. A large-button phone with a speed-dialing feature. A tub bench to help you take a bath or shower. Dressing sticks and reachers so you can groom yourself with ease. Canes, walkers, and motorized wheelchairs to help you get from place to place. The list of convenient appliances and tools is endless.

These environmental aids don't halt the progression of osteoarthritis. But they do help you become more productive, making your life more meaningful. Talk to your physician or a local home-health-care agency about where you can purchase these products.

Mind over Matter

What goes on in our heads has a lot to do with what goes on in our bodies. Your mood and emotion greatly influence your health, particularly the immune system. This mind/health link has been repeatedly demonstrated by scientific research over the past several decades.

Less clear is the specific role of the mind on the progression of degenerative joint disease. Increasingly though, psychiatric and psychological counseling is becoming a vital part of treatment plans for various illness. So it stands to reason that counseling can play a key role in treating osteoarthritis and other degenerative joint diseases.

Alternative Therapies: Some Unconventional Approaches

Don't scoff at the notion of alternative and unconventional treatments. At one time, arthroplasty (joint replacement) was considered an alternative treatment. Today, it's widely accepted.

Generally speaking, the treatments about to be discussed in this chapter aren't being used by conventional medical practitioners.

That's not to say they don't work or aren't useful. It just means they haven't been studied enough to reach any definite conclusions. Nor is there agreement about their usefulness.

By comparison, these treatments cost a lot less than conventional treatments. Considering how fast health-care costs are escalating, any less-expensive treatment deserves serious attention—much more than is being given at the moment. I believe that these treatments should be researched thoroughly in an unbiased manner. Unlike some conventional treatments, they're safe and free from unpleasant side effects. If effective, they could pay large dividends in reducing the long-term costs of treating osteoarthritis and other degenerative joint diseases. Table 13.1 (page 204) lists some of the more popular unconventional ways to treat degenerative joint diseases.

Healing Knowledge

■ The more you know, the better you can fight degenerative joint disease. If you know everything there is to know about your joints and how to take care of them, you're much more likely to prevent or recover from joint problems. With this book, my goal has been to educate as many people as possible about what degenerative joint disease is—and the new ways you can improve your treatment. That way, you can choose the best possible combination of treatments and side-step potential pitfalls, as long as you've educated yourself.

But education doesn't stop with you. Physicians and other health-care providers need continuing education to keep abreast of new developments as well. But often treatments can't keep pace with the progression of the disease. That's why patients must be taught to adjust their habits and lifestyle to compensate for their disabilities. Qualified, trained health-care professionals are in the best position to provide this level of education.

The treatment picture is constantly changing, too. Just think: Many of the treatment options available today were once studies in a research lab. Research offers real hope for a condition that has few total cures.

For now, prevention is the key. Take polio, for example. At one time, polio was a major health scourge, requiring considerable national resources to keep people alive. Then came the cure in the form of a vaccine for children. The prevention of millions of polio cases worldwide eradicated the need for expensive, long-term, and almost always unsuccessful treatment.

Today, arthritis is the leading disabler—a modern epidemic. But hopefully, with more research and education, it will go the way of other crippling diseases of the past.

UNCONVENTIONAL TREATMENTS FOR DEGENERATIVE JOINT DISEASES

Homeopathy

Auriculotherapy

Herbal Medicine

Naturopathy

Dietary Changes

Topical DMSO

Topical Capsaicin (Pepper)

TABLE 13.1

SUMMARY OF CONVENTIONAL TREATMENTS FOR DEGENERATIVE JOINT DISEASES*

Pharmacological (Drugs)

Oral

    Aspirin (salicylates)

    NSAIDs (ibuprofen, etc.)

    Acetaminophen (Tylenol)

    Other painkillers (codeine, propoxyphene)

    Muscle relaxants (for muscle spasms)

    Colchicine (rarely)

Injectable

    Corticosteroids (in joints)

    Anesthetics (lidocaine) (around and in joints)

Physical Medicine (Physical Therapy)

Biomechanical Interventions (traction, splints, orthotics, modified shoes, cervical collars, trusses)

Therapeutic Exercises

Reconstructive Therapy (Prolotherapy or Sclerotherapy)

Thermotherapy

Cryotherapy

Manipulative Therapies

Massage

Electrical Stimulation (TENS, etc.)

Surgery

Arthroscopy

Synovectomy

Tenotomy

Osteotomy (Bone removal to change joint geometry)

Resection (remove bad parts and reshape)

Implants

Arthroplasty (Joint replacement)

Arthrodesis (Joint fusion)

Environmental Aids

Canes, walkers, tub seats, toilet seats, button hooks, zipper hooks, car-door openers, motorized wheelchairs, etc.

Education

Patient Education

Vocational Training/Retraining

Physician Continuing Education

Research

Psychological Support

Counseling

....

Imaging

....

*NOTE: These treatments were listed in at least one of several authoritative medical textbooks on arthritis published since 1992.

TABLE 13.2

Epilogue

I hope you now have a better understanding of how specific nutrients (nutraceuticals) influence joint health. The research and case studies I've shared with you represent only a fraction of the existing information on nutrients and joint health. Even so, there's always room for more studies, especially with vitamin C and other supplemental nutrients.

Most of the nutrients discussed here work so well that they're actually drugs in other countries. Nutrients are remarkably safe, especially when you consider the side effects of drugs commonly used to treat joint disease.

Your body can heal itself, as long as it's well-stocked with the proper nutrients. Your body and its cells recognize these nutrients as part of themselves. They use those nutrients as both raw materials and as regulators of vital functions. Dr. Arnold Soren, a professor of orthopaedic surgery at New York University Medical Center in New York City, routinely gives his degenerative joint disease patients a multiple vitamin supplement to prevent further complications. He feels that the most important vitamins are vitamin C, D, and E, mostly for their roles in bones and non-cartilage joint tissues. Dr. Soren's work has been precedent-setting in the treatment of joint problems.

As you've seen, specific nutrients guard your joints from damage. They heal what might otherwise have been impossible to mend. Reversing the early stages of osteoarthritis is possible. So is cutting recovery time from injuries in half–as long as you use the right nutrients at the right time and in the right amounts. The protocols in this book tell you how.

I encourage you to work with your doctors. Standard therapies have much to offer for joint health and should never be ignored. Understand what these therapies are. Every doctor knows that a fully informed patient is a more cooperative patient. This attitude increases the chances for a better outcome. Also, the informed patient can better communicate with doctors. Scientific studies have shown repeatedly that patients who ask more questions and who are interested in their treatment recover faster than those who meekly submit to everything like sheep.

Use this book as a resource to educate both yourself and your doctors, particularly if they're unfamiliar with nutrients and joint health. Together, you and your doctors form a powerful fighting force against osteoarthritis and degenerative joint disease.

Glossary

Anatomy: the study of body structures.

Antioxidants: term used to describe different kinds of compounds that specifically neutralize free radicals, thereby protecting cells and tissues from damage.

Arthritis: generic term for the erosion or damage of joints.

Ascorbate: scientific name for vitamin C.

Biochemistry: the study of molecules used by and found in living things.

Bones: hard components of the skeleton. Bones provide attachments for muscles and joint structures so that movement can happen.

Bursae: fluid-filled sacs that act as ball bearings to allow easy sliding and gliding of tendons near joints.

Bursitis: inflammation of bursae. Overuse, improper motion, or physical damage to bursae can produce inflammation, resulting pain in and tenderness near joints.

Cartilage: tissue capping the ends of bones. Cartilage also forms structures of the ear and nose and makes up the discs in between bones of the spine. Cartilage absorbs shock and provides smooth surfaces for easy joint movement.

Chondrocytes: cells that live in and manufacture cartilage.

Chondroitin Sulfates: chondroprotective agent that is the most common glycosaminoglycan and major component of proteoglycans.

Chondroprotective agents: any substance (nutrient, drug, or hormone) that enhances the ability of joint cells to repair themselves.

Collagen: tough protein that makes up most body structures. It is the most abundant protein in human bodies.

Corticosteroids: type of hormone made from cholesterol produced by adrenal glands in response to stress. Both nature-identical and synthetic corticosteroids have been extensively used to reduce inflammation. Like all powerful agents, corticosteroids are toxic with long-term use.

Crepitus: creaking, crackling, or rubbing noises heard in joints during movement.

Cytokine: small protein or other molecule produced by cells to affect actions in neighboring cells. Cytokines can trigger many cell responses and are very powerful regulators of what cells do.

Degenerative Joint Disease: any number of conditions or diseases that result in deterioration of cartilage and loss of joint functions.

Dietitian: person (usually registered and licensed) who has studied and now applies dietetics to improve the health of people.

Dietetics: the study of foods and how to feed people for medical purposes.

Eicosanoids: scientific term for the tiny molecules produced by most cells from certain fats (like omega-3 oils) that are very powerful regulators of cell functions. Like cytokines, eicosanoids can greatly influence what cells do.

Elastin: protein similar to collagen, but arranged like a net or web instead of a rope. In this way, elastin can stretch and spring back to its original shape.

Inflammation: response of tissues to injury or damage. There are two kinds of inflammation—acute and chronic. Inflammation is characterized by heat, swelling, pain, redness, and loss of function. If prolonged, too much inflammation can delay healing.

Fibroblast: cells that live in and manufacture and repair most connective tissues.

Free Radicals: very reactive molecules formed by normal cell processes or pollution. Free radicals damage cell components, unless stopped by antioxidants.

Glucosamine: chondroprotective agent that regulates cartilage synthesis.

Glycosaminoglycans (GAGs): several types of long chains composed of modified sugars and usually containing sulfur. Hyaluronan and chondroitin sulfates are most important GAGs to joints.

Glycosylation: process of adding sugars to proteins or to each other in long chains.

Hyaluronan: a very long chain of glucosamine and another modified sugar (no sulfur). Hyaluronan forms the backbone for proteoglycans and gives lubricating properties for synovial fluid. Hyaluronan is also a chondroprotective agent licensed as a drug for veterinary use.

Intervertebral Disc: large disc-shaped piece of special cartilage between vertebra in the spine. Like joint cartilage, discs can degenerate, causing low back pain or neck pain.

Ischemia: low oxygen levels in tissues.

Joint: the body structure where two bone ends meet.

Ligaments: tough but slightly elastic connectors of bone to bone.

Low-Back Pain: pain in lower back area caused by degeneration of invertebral discs, bony overgrowth, osteoarthritic changes. Nerves are squeezed, causing pain. Low back pain includes sciatica, which is pain in the leg.

Lymphatics: separate circulatory system of vessels that reaches most body areas. This system contains lymph fluid and immune system cells. Lymphatics drain into lymph nodes and eventually, the bloodstream.

Lymphocytes: one type of white blood cell. Different kinds of lymphocytes produce antibodies (B cells), control other immune system cells (T helper cells, T suppressor cells), or kill foreign cells (Natural Killer cells). Lymphocytes are an essential cell type for life.

Meniscus: menisci (plural form of meniscus) are the washers of the human body and are found inside of major joints, especially the knee joint. Menisci are made of specialized cartilage. Menisci can be damaged, leading to frequent removal. Premature arthritis usually accompanies meniscus removal.

Metabolism: process by which the body converts foods into energy and body structures.

Musculoskeletal system: combined tissues that give us shape, support other organs, and generate movement. The musculoskeletal system includes muscles, bones and joints.

Niacinamide: scientific name for vitamin B3. A chondroprotective agent.

NSAIDs: NSAIDs is an abbreviation for non-steroidal anti-inflammatory drugs. Several types of chemicals are NSAIDs, but all have effects on reducing inflammation and pain by knocking out prostaglandins (both good and bad ones). Some NSAIDs in high doses may prevent repair of cartilage. Common NSAIDs include aspirin, acetaminophen, and ibuprofen.

Nutrition: the study of what we eat and how it becomes part of us. Nutrition includes many scientific fields, including anatomy, physiology, biochemistry, enzymology, pharmacokinetics, psychology, dietetics, anthropology and others.

Nutritionist: term describing a wide variety of individuals (some certified and some not) who concern themselves with people's health by counseling what to eat.

Osteoarthritis (OA): one of the two major types of arthritis. Osteoarthritis is the slow, gradual erosion of cartilage, accompanied by bony overgrowth, until pain and loss of function appears.

Osteocytes: cells that live in and maintain bone.

Osteoporosis: bone loss, especially in women after menopause.

Physiology: the study of how the body works.

Prostaglandins: another, older name for eicosanoids.

Proteoglycans: combination of protein and many long chains of modified sugars, usually containing sulfur. They are found everywhere in the body, especially in cartilage. Proteoglycans form a stiff gel to resist compression.

Proteoglycan Subunits: consist of a core protein with several hundred glycosaminoglycan chains attached. Produced by chondrocytes, proteoglycan subunits assemble into large proteoglycans.

Retinol: scientific name for vitamin A. Retinol is not beta carotene.

Rheumatism: another name for rheumatoid arthritis (see rheumatoid arthritis).

Rheumatoid Arthritis (RA): one of the two major types of arthritis. Rheumatoid arthritis is also called inflammatory arthritis and is associated with immune system involvement. Joint pain, swelling, and damage are accompanied by other symptoms like fatigue and fever. Rheumatoid arthritis may come and go.

Subchondral bone: the bone just underneath cartilage that is slightly spongy. It can absorb shocks and contains blood vessels that deliver oxygen and nutrients to cartilage.

Synovial Fluid: slippery fluid inside joint cavities that reduces friction in joints. This fluid is comprised mostly of hyaluronan with some blood plasma.

Synoviocytes: cells in the synovium. They secrete synovial joint fluid (hyaluronan) to reduce joint friction, but also produce regulatory molecules that may contribute to arthritis.

Synovium: tissue that lines the inside of joints. Synovium contains several cell layers with blood vessels, nerves and lymphatics that help nourish joints.

Tendinitis: inflammation around tendons near joints. Also called tenosynovitis.

Tendons: strong rope-like or flat bundles of collagen that connect muscles to bone.

Tocopherols: scientific name for vitamin E.

REFERENCES

PART I

CHAPTER 1:
WHAT KIND OF ARTHRITIS DO YOU HAVE?

Alarcón, G. S. "Seronegative Polyarthritis," Chapter 56 in *Arthritis and Allied Conditions. A Textbook of Rheumatology*, Vol. 1, 12th ed., D. J. McCarty, W. J. Koopman, eds., Philadelphia: Lea and Febiger, 1993, 1013-1020.

Altman, R. D., Howell D. S., Gottlieb N. L. "New Directions in Therapy of Osteoarthritis," *Sem. Arth. Rheum.*, 1987; 17(Suppl. 1):1-2.

Ball, G. V. "Ankylosing Spondylitis," Chapter 59 in *Arthritis and Allied Conditions. A Textbook of Rheumatology*, Vol. 1, 12th ed., D. J. McCarty, W. J. Koopman, eds., Philadelphia: Lea and Febiger, 1993, 1051-1060.

Bennett, R. M. "Psoriatic Arthritis," Chapter 61 in *Arthritis and Allied Conditions. A Textbook of Rheumatology*, Vol. 1, 12th ed., D. J. McCarty, W. J. Koopman, eds., Philadelphia: Lea and Febiger, 1993, 1079-1094.

Bland, J. H., and S.M. Cooper. "Osteoarthritis: A Review of the Cell Biology Involved and Evidence for Reversibility. Management Rationally Related to Known Genesis and Pathophysiology," *Sem. Arth. Rheum.*, 1984; 14: 106-133.

Bucci, L. R. "Reversal of Osteoarthritis by Nutritional Intervention," *Am. Chiropractic Assoc. J. of Chiropractic*, 1990; 27(11):69-72.

Bucci, L. R. "Chondroprotective Agents. Glucosamine Salts and Chondroitin Sulfates," *Townsend Letter for Doctors*, 1994; 124:52-54.

Bucci, L. R. *Nutrition Applied to Injury Rehabilitation and Sports Medicine*, Boca Raton, Florida: CRC Press, 1994.

Bullough, P. G. "The Pathology of Osteoarthritis," Chapter 3 in *Osteoarthritis. Diagnosis and Medical/Surgical Management*, 2nd ed., R. W. Moskowitz, D. S. Howell, V. M. Goldberg,

H. J. Mankin, eds., Philadelphia: W. B. Saunders, 1992, 39-69.

Cush, J. J., P. E. Lipsky. "Reiter's Syndrome and Reactive Arthritis," Chapter 60 in *Arthritis and Allied Conditions. A Textbook of Rheumatology*, Vol. 1, 12th ed., D. J. McCarty, W. J. Koopman, eds., Philadelphia: Lea and Febiger, 1993, 1,061-1,078.

Dieppe, P., and J. M. Rogers. "Skeletal Paleopathology of Rheumatic Diseases," Chapter 2 in *Arthritis and Allied Conditions. A Textbook of Rheumatology*, Vol. 1, 12th ed., D. J. McCarty, W. J. Koopman, eds., Philadelphia: Lea and Febiger, 1993, 9-16.

Espinoza, L. R. "Retrovirus-Associated Rheumatic Syndromes," Chapter 122 in *Arthritis and Allied Conditions. A Textbook of Rheumatology*, Vol. 2, 12th ed., D. J. McCarty, W. J. Koopman, eds., Philadelphia: Lea and Febiger, 1993, 2,087-2,100.

Felson, D. T. "Epidemiology of the Rheumatic Diseases," Chapter 3 in *Arthritis and Allied Conditions. A Textbook of Rheumatology*, Vol. 1, 12th ed., D. J. McCarty, W. J. Koopman, eds., Philadelphia: Lea and Febiger, 1993, 17-48.

Fife, R. S. "A Short History of Osteoarthritis," Chapter 1 in *Osteoarthritis. Diagnosis and Medical/Surgical Management*, 2nd ed., R. W. Moskowitz, D. S. Howell, V. M. Goldberg, H. J. Mankin, eds., Philadelphia: W. B. Saunders, 1992, 11-14.

Ghosh, P., and P. Brooks. "Chondroprotection–Exploring the Concept," *J. Rheumatol.*, 1991; 18:161-166.

Goldenberg, D. L. "Gonococcal Arthritis and Other Neisserial Infections," Chapter 117 in *Arthritis and Allied Conditions. A Textbook of Rheumatology*, Vol. 2, 12th ed., D. J. McCarty, W. J. Koopman, eds., Philadelphia: Lea and Febiger, 1993, 2,025-2,034.

Goldenberg, D. L. "Bacterial Arthritis," Chapter 27 in *Arthritis Surgery*, C. B. Sledge, S. Ruddy, E. D. Harris, W. N. Kelley, eds., Philadelphia: W. B. Saunders, 1994, 495-512.

Ho, G. "Bacterial Arthritis," Chapter 116 in *Arthritis and Allied Conditions. A Textbook of Rheumatology*, Vol. 2, 12th ed., D. J. McCarty, W. J. Koopman, eds., Philadelphia: Lea and Febiger, 1993, 2,003-2,024.

Mankin, H. J. "Clinical Features of Osteoarthritis," Chapter 25 in *Osteoarthritis. Diagnosis and Medical/Surgical Management*, 2nd ed., R. W. Moskowitz, D. S. Howell, V. M. Goldberg, H. J. Mankin, eds., Philadelphia: W. B. Saunders, 1992, 469-479.

McCarty, D. J. "Differential Diagnosis of Arthritis: Analysis of Signs and Symptoms," Chapter 4 in *Arthritis and Allied Conditions. A Textbook of Rheumatology*, Vol. 1, 12th ed., D. J. McCarty, W. J. Koopman, eds., Philadelphia: Lea and Febiger, 1993, 49-61.

McCarty, D. J. "Clinical Picture of Rheumatoid Arthritis," Chapter 43 in *Arthritis and Allied Conditions. A Textbook of Rheumatology*, Vol. 1, 12th ed., D. J. McCarty, W. J. Koopman, eds., Philadelphia: Lea and Febiger, 1993, 781-809.

McCarty, D. J., and W. J. Koopman, eds., Section VI. "Systemic Rheumatic Diseases," Chapters 66-88 in *Arthritis and Allied Conditions. A Textbook of Rheumatology*, Vol. 2, 12th ed., D. J. McCarty, W. J. Koopman, eds., Philadelphia: Lea and Febiger, 1993, 1,149-1,517.

Meier, J. L., and G. S. Hoffman. "Mycobacterial and Fungal Infections," Chapter 28 in *Arthritis Surgery*, C. B. Sledge, S. Ruddy, E. D. Harris, W. N. Kelley, eds., Philadelphia: W. B. Saunders, 1994, 513-529.

Messner, R. P. "Arthritis Due to Mycobacteria, Fungi and Parasites," Chapter 118 in *Arthritis and Allied Conditions. A Textbook of Rheumatology*, Vol. 2, 12th ed., D. J. McCarty, W. J. Koopman, eds., Philadelphia: Lea and Febiger, 1993, 2,035-2,046.

Mielants, H., and E. M. Veys. "Enteropathic Arthritis," Chapter 62 in *Arthritis and Allied Conditions. A Textbook of Rheumatology*, Vol. 1, 12th ed., D. J. McCarty, W. J. Koopman, eds.,

Philadelphia: Lea and Febiger, 1993, 1,095-1,109.

Moskowitz, R. W. Introduction in *Osteoarthritis. Diagnosis and Medical/Surgical Management*, 2nd ed., R. W. Moskowitz, D. S. Howell, V. M. Goldberg, H. J. Mankin, eds., Philadelphia: W. B. Saunders, 1992, 1-7.

Moskowitz, R. W. "Clinical and Laboratory Findings in Osteoarthritis," Chapter 103 in *Arthritis and Allied Conditions. A Textbook of Rheumatology*, Vol. 2, 12th ed., D. J. McCarty, W. J. Koopman, eds., Philadelphia: Lea and Febiger, 1993, 1,735-1,760.

Pachman, L. M., and A.K. Poznanski. "Juvenile Rheumatoid Arthritis," Chapter 57 in *Arthritis and Allied Conditions. A Textbook of Rheumatology*, Vol. 1, 12th ed., D. J. McCarty, W. J. Koopman, eds., Philadelphia: Lea and Febiger, 1993, 1,021-1,038.

Peyron, J. G., and R. D. Altman. "The Epidemiology of Osteoarthritis," Chapter 2 in *Osteoarthritis. Diagnosis and Medical/Surgical Management*, 2nd ed., R. W. Moskowitz, D. S. Howell, V. M. Goldberg, H. J. Mankin, eds., Philadelphia: W. B. Saunders, 1992, 15-37.

Radin, E.L., and D. B. Burr. "Hypothesis: Joints Can Heal," *Sem. Arth. Rheum.*, 1984; 13:293-302.

Rahn, D. W., and S. E. Malawista. "Lyme Disease," Chapter 120 in *Arthritis and Allied Conditions. A Textbook of Rheumatology*, Vol. 2, 12th ed., D. J. McCarty, W. J. Koopman, eds., Philadelphia: Lea and Febiger, 1993, 2,067-2,079.

Reimann, I., S. B. Christensen, and N. H. Diemer. "Observations of Reversibility of Glycosaminoglycan Depletion in Articular Cartilage," *Clin. Orthop.*, 1982; 168:258-264.

Rothschild, B. M. "Skeletal Paleopathology of Rheumatic Diseases: The Subhomo Connection," Chapter 1 in *Arthritis and Allied Conditions. A Textbook of Rheumatology*, Vol. 1, 12th ed., D. J. McCarty, W. J. Koopman, eds., Philadelphia: Lea and Febiger, 1993, 3-8.

Schmid, F. R. "Principles of Diagnosis and Treatment of Bone and Joint Infections," Chapter 115 in *Arthritis and Allied Conditions. A Textbook of Rheumatology*, Vol. 2, 12th ed., D. J. McCarty, W. J. Koopman, eds., Philadelphia: Lea and Febiger, 1993, 1,975-2,002.

Upchurch, K. A., and D. B. Brettler. "Hemophilic arthropath," Chapter 29 in *Arthritis Surgery*, C. B. Sledge, S. Ruddy, E. D. Harris, W. N. Kelley, eds., Philadelphia: W. B. Saunders, 1994, 530-539.

Ytterberg, S. R. "Viral Arthritis," Chapter 119 in *Arthritis and Allied Conditions. A Textbook of Rheumatology*, Vol. 2, 12th ed., D. J. McCarty, W. J. Koopman, eds., Philadelphia: Lea and Febiger, 1993, 2,047-2,066.

CHAPTER 2:

WHAT YOU DON'T KNOW ABOUT YOUR JOINTS CAN HURT YOU

Adolphe, M., Ed., *Biological Regulation of the Chondrocytes*, Boca Raton, Florida: CRC Press, 1992.

American Academy of Orthopedic Surgeons, "The Musculoskeletal System," Chapter 13, in *Athletic Training and Sports Medicine*, 2nd ed., Park Ridge, Illinois: Park American Academy of Orthopedic Surgeons, 1991, 192-202.

Buckwalter, J. A., L. C. Rosenberg, and E. B. Hunziker. "Articular Cartilage: Composition, Structure, Response to Injury, and Methods of Facilitating Repair," in *Articular Cartilage and Knee Joint Function*, Ewing, J. W., Ed., New York: Raven Press, 1990, 19-38.

Coe, F. L., and M. J. Favus, eds., *Disorders of Bone and Mineral Metabolism*, New York: Raven Press, 1992.

Freeman, M. A. R., Ed., *Adult Articular Cartilage*, 2nd ed., Kent, England: Pittman Medical Publishing, 1979.

Gamble, J. G., Ed., *The Musculoskeletal System. Physiological Basics*, New York: Raven, 1988.

Ghadially, F. N. *Fine Structure of Synovial Joints*, London: Butterworths, 1983.

Henderson, B., and J. C. W. Edwards. *The Synovial Lining in Health and Disease*, London: Chapman and Hill, 1987.

Kucharz, E. J. *The Collagens: Biochemistry and Pathophysiology*, Berlin: Springer-Verlag, 1992.

Kuettner, K. E., R. Schleyerbach, and V. C. Hascall, eds., *Articular Cartilage Biochemistry*, New York: Raven Press, 1985.

Kuhn, K., and T. Krieg, eds., *Connective Tissue: Biological and Clinical Aspects*, Vol. 10, in *Rheumatology. An Annual Review*, Schattenkirchner, M., Ed. Basel, Switzerland: Karger, 1986.

Mankin, H. J., and E. L. Radin. "Structure and Function of Joints," Chapter 9 in *Arthritis and Allied Conditions. A Textbook of Rheumatology*, Vol. 1, D. J. McCarty, W. J. Koopman, eds., Philadelphia: Lea and Febiger, 1993, 181-198.

Marieb, E. N. "Tissues: The Living Fabric," Chapter 4 in *Human Anatomy and Physiology*, Redwood City, California: Benjamin/Cummings Publishing Co., 1989, 100-132.

McCarty, D. J., and W. J. Koopman, eds., *Arthritis and Allied Conditions. A Textbook of Rheumatology*. Vol. 2, 12th ed., Philadelphia: Lea and Febiger, 1993.

McLatchie, G. R., C. M. E. Lennox, E. C. Percy, and J. Davies, eds., *The Soft Tissues. Trauma and Sports Injuries*, Oxford: Butterworth-Heinemann, 1993.

Nimni, M. E., and B. R. Olsen, eds., *Collagen*, Vols. I-IV, Boca Raton, Florida: CRC Press, 1988, 1989.

Norkin, C. C., and P. K. Levangie, eds., *Joint Structure and Function. A Comprehensive Analysis*, 2nd ed., Philadelphia: F. A. Davis, 1992.

Norris, C. M. *Sports Injuries. Diagnosis and Management for Physiotherapists*, Oxford: Butterworth-Heinemann, 1993.

Parks, R. M. "Lower Extremity Sports Injuries," Chapter 5 in *Sports and Exercise Medicine*, S.C. Wood, R. C. Roach, eds., New York: Marcel Dekker, 1994.

Renström, P. A. F. H., Ed., *Sports Injuries. Basic Principles of Prevention and Care*, Oxford: Blackwell Scientific Publications, 1993.

Robert, L., W. Hornebeck, eds., *Elastin and Elastases*, Vols. I and II, Boca Raton, Florida: CRC Press, 1989.

Rosse, C., and G. K. Clawson, eds., *The Musculoskeletal System in Health and Disease*, Hagerstown, Pennsylvania: Harper and Row, 1980.

Silver, F. H. *Biological Materials: Structure, Mechanical Properties, and Modeling of Soft Tissues*, New York: New York University Press, 1987.

Sledge, C. B. "Biology of the Joint," Chapter 1 in *Arthritis Surgery*, C. B. Sledge, S. Ruddy, E. D. Harris, W. N. Kelley, eds., Philadelphia: W.B. Saunders, 1994, 1-21.

Sokoloff, L., Ed., *The Joints and Synovial Fluid*, Vol. 2, Academic Press, 1980.

Trelstad, R. L., and P. D. Kemp. "Matrix Glycoproteins and Proteoglycans," Chapter 4 in *Arthritis Surgery*, C. B. Sledge, S. Ruddy, E. D. Harris, W. N. Kelley, eds., Philadelphia: W. B. Saunders, 1994, 48-70.

Varma, R. S., and R. Varma, eds., *Glycosaminoglycans and Proteoglycans in Physiological and Pathological Processes of Body Systems,* Basel, Switzerland: Karger, 1982.

Wight, T. N., and R. P. Mecham, eds., *Biology of the Proteoglycans,* Orlando: Academic Press, 1987.

Wilson, F. C., Ed., *The Musculoskeletal System. Basic Processes and Disorders,* 2nd ed., Philadelphia: Lippincott, 1983.

CHAPTER 3:
OSTEOARTHRITIS: ARE YOU AT RISK?

Altman, R. D., D. S. Howell, and N. L. Gottlieb. "New Directions in Therapy of Osteoarthritis," *Sem. Arth. Rheum.,* 1987; 17(Suppl. 1):1-2.

Bland, J. H., and S. M. Cooper. "Osteoarthritis: A Review of the Cell Biology Involved and Evidence for Reversibility. Management Rationally Related to Known Genesis and Pathophysiology," *Sem. Arth. Rheum.,* 1984; 14: 106-133.

Brandt, K. D. and H. J. Mankin. "Pathogenesis of Osteoarthritis," Chapter 24 in *Arthritis Surgery,* C. B. Sledge, S. Ruddy, S. D. Harris, W. N. Kelley, eds. Philadelphia: W. B. Saunders, 1994, 450-468.

Bucci, L. R. "Reversal of Osteoarthritis by Nutritional Intervention," *Am. Chiropractic Assoc. J. of Chiropractic,* 1990; 27(11):69-72.

Bucci, L. R. "Chondroprotective Agents. Glucosamine Salts and Chondroitin Sulfates," *Townsend Letter for Doctors,* 1994; 124:52-54.

Bucci, L. R. *Nutrition Applied to Injury Rehabilitation and Sports Medicine,* Boca Raton, Florida: CRC Press, 1994.

Dieppe, P., and J. Cunningham. "The Natural Course and Prognosis of Osteoarthritis," Chapter 17 in *Osteoarthritis. Diagnosis and Medical/Surgical Management,* 2nd Ed., R. W. Moskowitz, D. S. Howell, V. M. Goldberg, and H. J. Mankin, eds., Philadelphia: W. B. Saunders, 1992, 399-412.

Ghosh, P., and P. Brooks. "Chondroprotection–Exploring the Concept," *J. Rheumatol.,* 1991; 18:161-166.

Hough, A. J. "Pathology of Osteoarthritis," Chapter 101 in *Arthritis and Allied Conditions. A Textbook of Rheumatology,* Vol. 2, 12th Ed., D. J. McCarty, W. J. Koopman, eds. Philadelphia: Lea and Febiger, 1993, 1,699-1,721.

Jones, J. P. "Osteonecrosis," Chapter 100 in *Arthritis and Allied Conditions. A Textbook of Rheumatology,* Vol. 2, 12th Ed., D. J. McCarty, W. J. Koopman, eds. Philadelphia: Lea and Febiger, 1993, 1,677-1,696.

Moskowitz, R. W. "Clinical and Laboratory Findings in Osteoarthritis," Chapter 103 in *Arthritis and Allied Conditions. A Textbook of Rheumatology,* Vol. 2, 12th Ed., D. J. McCarty, W. J. Koopman, eds. Philadelphia: Lea and Febiger, 1993, 1,735-1,760.

Moskowitz, R. W., D. S. Howell, V. M. Goldberg, and H. J. Mankin, eds. *Osteoarthritis. Diagnosis and Medical/Surgical Management,* 2nd Ed. Philadelphia: W. B. Saunders, 1992.

Pinals, R. S. "Traumatic Arthritis and Allied Conditions," Chapter 89 in *Arthritis and Allied Conditions. A Textbook of Rheumatology,* Vol. 2, 12th Ed., D. J. McCarty, W. J. Koopman, eds. Philadelphia: Lea and Febiger, 1993, 1,521-1,537.

Radin, E. L., and D. B. Burr. "Hypothesis: Joints Can Heal," *Sem. Arth. Rheum.,* 1984; 13:293-302.

Reimann, I., S. B. Christensen, and N. H. Diemer. "Observations of Reversibility of Glycosaminoglycan Depletion in Articular Cartilage," *Clin. Orthop.*, 1982; 168:258-264.

Rothschild, B. M. "Skeletal Paleopathology of Rheumatic Diseases: The Subhomo Connection," Chapter 1 in *Arthritis and Allied Conditions. A Textbook of Rheumatology*, Vol. 1, 12th ed., D. J. McCarty, W. J. Koopman, eds., Philadelphia: Lea and Febiger, 1993, 3-8.

Schumacher, H. R. "Secondary Osteoarthritis," Chapter 16 in *Osteoarthritis. Diagnosis and Medical/Surgical Management*, 2nd Ed. Philadelphia: W. B. Saunders, 1992, 367-398.

PART II

....

CHAPTER 4:
GLUCOSAMINES: THE KEY BREAKTHROUGH FOR JOINT HEALTH

Böhmer, D., P. Ambrus, A. Szögy, and G. Haralambie. "Treatment of Chondropathia Patellae in Young Athletes with Glucosamine Sulfate," in *Current Topics in Sports Medicine*, N. Bachl, L. Prokop, and R. Suckert, eds., Vienna: Urban and Schwarzenberg, 1984, 799-803.

Bucci, L. R. "Reversal of Osteoarthritis by Nutritional Intervention," *Am. Chiropractic Assoc. J. of Chiropractic*, 1990; 27(11):69-72.

Bucci, L. R. "Chondroprotective Agents. Glucosamine Salts and Chondroitin Sulfates," *Townsend Letter for Doctors*, 1994; 124:52-54.

Bucci, L. R. *Nutrition Applied to Injury Rehabilitation and Sports Medicine*, Boca Raton, Florida: CRC Press, 1994.

Crolle, G., and E. D'Este. "Glucosamine Sulfate for the Management of Arthrosis: A Controlled Clinical Investigation," *Curr. Res. Med. Opinion*, 1980; 7(2):104-109.

D'Ambrosio, E., B. Casa, R. Bompani, G. Scali, and M. Scali. "Glucosamine Sulphate: A Controlled Clinical Investigation in Arthrosis," *Pharmatherapeutica*, 1981; 2(8):504-508.

Drovanti, A., A. A. Bignamini, and A. L. Rovati. "Therapeutic Activity of Oral Glucosamine Sulfate in Osteoarthritis: A Placebo-Controlled Double-Blind Investigation," *Clin. Ther.*, 1980; 3(4):260-272.

Karzel, K., and R. Domenjoz. "Effects of Hexosamine Derivatives and Uronic Acid Derivatives on Glycosaminoglycan Metabolism of Fibroblast Cultures," *Pharmacology*, 1971; 5:337-345.

Prudden, J. F., P. Migel, P. Hanson, L. Friedrich, and L. Balassa. "The Discovery of a Potent Pure Chemical Wound-Healing Accelerator," *Am. J. Surg.*, 1970; 119:560-564.

Pujalte, J. M., E. P. Llavore, and F. R. Ylescupidez. "Double-Blind Clinical Evaluation of Oral Glucosamine Sulphate in the Basic Treatment of Osteoarthrosis," *Curr. Res. Med. Opinion*, 1980; 7(2):110-114.

Rodén, L. "Effect of Hexosamines on the Synthesis of Chondroitin Sulphuric Acid in Vitro," *Ark. Kemi.*, 1956; 10:345-352.

Setnikar, I., C. Giachetti, and G. Zanolo. "Absorption, Distribution and Excretion of Radioactivity After a Single Intravenous or Oral Administration of [^{14}C] Glucosamine to the Rat," *Pharmatherapeutica*, 1984; 3(8):538-550.

Setnikar, I., C. Giacchetti, and G. Zanolo. "Pharmacokinetics of Glucosamine in the Dog and Man," *Arzneim. Forsch.*, 1986; 36(2):729-736.

Setnikar, I., R. Cereda, M. A. Pacini, and L. Revel. "Antireactive Properties of Glucosamine Sulfate," *Arzneim. Forsch.*, 1991; 41(2):157-161.

Setnikar, I., M. A. Pacini, and L. Revel. "Antiarthritic Effects of Glucosamine Sulfate Studied in Animal Models," *Arzneim. Forsch.*, 1991; 41(5):542-545.

Tapadinhas, M. J., I. C. Rivera, and A. A. Bignamini. "Oral Glucosamine Sulphate in the Management of Arthrosis: Report on a Multi-Centre Open Investigation in Portugal," *Pharmatherapeutica*, 1982; 3(3):157-168.

Tesoriere, G., F. Dones, D. Magistro, and L. Castagnetta. "Intestinal Absorption of Glucosamine and N-Acetylglucosamine," *Experentia*, 1972; 28(7):770-771.

Vajaradul, Y. "Double-Blind Clinical Evaluation of Intra-Articular Glucosamine in Outpatients with Gonarthrosis," *Clin. Ther.*, 1981; 3(5):336-343.

Vaz, A. L. "Double-Blind Clinical Evaluation of the Relative Efficacy of Ibuprofen and Glucosamine Sulphate in the Management of Osteoarthrosis of the Knee in Out-Patients," *Curr. Med. Res. Opinion*, 1982; 8(3):145-149.

Vidal y Plana, R. R., D. Bizzarri, and A. L. Rovati. "Articular Cartilage Pharmacology: I. In Vitro Studies on Glucosamine and Non Steroidal Antiinflammatory Drugs," *Pharm. Res. Comm.*, 1978; 10(6):557-569.

CHAPTER 5:
ON THE MEND WITH "CHONDROPROTECTION"

Altman, R. D., and P. Kapila, D. D. Dean, and D. S. Howell. "Future Therapeutic Trends in Osteoarthritis," *Scand. J. Rheumatol. Suppl.*, 1988; 77:37-42.

Bird, H. "The Current Treatment of Osteoarthritis," Chapter 17 in *Osteoarthritis. Current Research and Prospects for Pharmacological Intervention*, R. G. G. Russell, and P. A. Dieppe, eds., London: I. B. C. Technical Services, Ltd., 1991, 173-196.

Bucci, L. R. "Reversal of Osteoarthritis by Nutritional Intervention," *A.C.A. J. Chiropractic*, 1990; 27(11):69-72.

Bucci, L. R. "Chondroprotective Agents. Glucosamine Salts and Chondroitin Sulfates," *Townsend Letter for Doctors*, 1994; 124:52-54.

Bucci, L. R. *Nutrition Applied to Injury Rehabilitation and Sports Medicine*, Boca Raton, Florida: CRC Press, 1994.

Burkhardt, D., and P. Ghosh. "Laboratory Evaluation of Glycosaminoglycan Polysulphate Ester for Chondroprotective Activity: A Review," *Curr. Ther. Res.*, 1986; 40(6):1,034-1,053.

Burkhardt D., and P. Ghosh. "Laboratory Evaluation of Antiarthritic Drugs as Potential Chondroprotective Agents," *Sem. Arth. Rheum.*, 1987; 17(2)Suppl.1:3-34.

Dinkel, R. "Der Okonomische Nutzen der Langzeitbehandlung von Coxarthrose-Patienten mit Arumalon," *Akt. Rheumatol.*, 1984; 9:149-152.

Dixon, A. S., R. K. Jacoby, H. Berry, and E. B. D. Hamilton. "Clinical Trial of Intra-Articular Injection of Sodium Hyaluronate in Patients with Osteoarthritis of the Knee," *Curr. Med. Res. Opin.*, 1988; 11:205-213.

Ghosh, P. "Anti-Rheumatic Drugs and Cartilage," *Baillieres Clin. Rheumatol.*, 1988; 2(2):309-338.

Ghosh, P., M. Smith, and C. Wells. "Second-Line Agents in Osteoarthritis," Chapter 15 in *Second-Line Agents in the Treatment of Rheumatic Diseases*, J. S. Dixon, and D. E. Furst, eds., New York: Marcel Dekker, 1992, 363-427.

Hess, H., and W. Thiel. "The Treatment of Posttraumatic Cartilage Damages by Intra-Articular Injections," in *Current Topics in Sports Medicine*, N. Bachl, L. Prokop, and R. Suckert, eds., Vienna: Urban and Schwarzenberg, 1984, 794-799.

Jimenez, R. "Innovative Therapeutic Agents," Chapter 6 in *Therapeutic Controversies in the Rheumatic Diseases*, R. F. Wilkens, and S. L. Dahl, eds., Orlando: Grune and Stratton, 1987, 213-251.

Kerzberg, E. M., E. J. A. Roldan, G. Castelli, and E. D. Huberman. "Combination of Glycosaminoglycans and Acetylsalicylic Acid in Knee Osteoarthritis," *Scand. J. Rheum.*, 1987; 16:377-380.

Kvist, M., M. Jarvinen, U. Kujala, B. Forsskahl. "Comparison of Arteparon and Indomethacin in the Treatment of Apicites Patellae and Peritendinitis of Ligamentum Patellae in Athletes," in *Current Topics in Sports Medicine*, N. Bachl, L. Prokop, and R. Suckert, eds., Vienna: Urban and Schwarzenberg, 1984, 825-835.

Leardini, G., A. Perbellini, M. Franceschini, and L. Mattara. "Intra-Articular Injections of Hyaluronic Acid in the Treatment of Painful Shoulder," *Clin. Ther.*, 1988; 10(5):521-525.

Lysholm, J. "The Relation Between Pain and Torque in an Isokinetic Strength Test of Knee Extension," *Arthroscopy*, 1987; 3(3):182-184.

Maier, R., and G. Wilhelmi. "Influence of Anti-Inflammatory Drugs on Spontaneous Osteoarthrosis in Mice," in *A New Antirheumatic-analgesic Agent: Pirprofen (Rengasil®)*, J. K. van der Korst, Ed., Bern: Hans Huber Publishers, 1979, 87-96.

Morrison, L. M., and N. L. Enrick. "Coronary Heart Disease: Reduction of Death Rate by Chondroitin Sulfate A," *Angiology*, 1973; 24:269-276.

Morrison L. M., and O. A. Schjeide. *Coronary Heart Disease and the Mucopolysaccharides (Glycosaminoglycans)*, Springfield, Illinois: C. C. Thomas, 1974.

Morrison, L. M. "Therapeutic Applications of Chondroitin-4-Sulfate. Appraisal of Biological Properties," *Folia Angiol.*, 1977; 25:225-231.

Morrison, L. M., and O. A. Schjeide. *Arteriosclerosis. Prevention, Treatment, and Regression*, Springfield, Illinois: C. C. Thomas, 1984.

Oliviero, U., G. P. Sorrentino, P. DePaola, E. Tranfaglia, A. D'Alessandr., S. Carifi, F. A. Porfido, R. Cerio, A. M. Grasso, and D. Policicchio. "Effects of the Treatment with Matrix on Elderly People with Chronic Articular Degeneration," *Drugs Exp. Clin. Res.*, 1991; 17(1):45-51.

Peliskova, Z., K. Trnavsky, and J. Krajickova-Trnavska. "The Present State of Chondroprotective Therapy in Osteoarthrosis," *Acta Chir. Orthop. Traumatol. Cech.*, 1989; 56:185-189.

Pinals, R. S. "Pharmacologic Treatment of Osteoarthritis," *Clin. Ther.*, 1992; 14(3):336-347.

Pipitone, V. R. "Chondroprotection with Chondroitin Sulfate," *Drugs Exp. Clin. Res.*, 1991; 17(1):3-7.

Prino, G. "Pharmacological Profile of Ateroid," *Mod. Probl. Pharmacopsychiatry*, 1989; 23:68-74.

Prudden, J. F., and J. Allen. "The Clinical Acceleration of Healing with a Cartilage Preparation, a Controlled Study," *JAMA*, 1965; 192(5): 352-354.

Prudden, J. F., and L. L. Balassa. "The Biological Activity of Bovine Cartilage Preparations," *Sem. Arth. Rheum.*, 1974; 3(4):287-321.

Rejholec, V. "Long-Term Studies of Antiosteoarthritic Drugs: An Assessment," *Sem. Arth. Rheum.*, 1987; 17(2)Suppl.1:35-53.

Santini, V. "A General Practice Trial of Ateroid 200 in 8,776 Patients with Chronic Senile Cerebral Insufficiency," *Mod. Probl. Pharmacopsychiatry*, 1989; 23:95-101.

Shichikawa, K., M. Igarashi, S. Sugawara, and Y. Iwasaki. "Clinical Evaluation of High Molecular Weight Sodium Hyaluronate (SPH) on Osteoarthritis of the Knee." Multicenter Well Controlled Study, *Rinsho Yakuri*, 1983; 14:545-558.

Sprengel, H., J. Franke, and A. Sprengel. "Personal Experiences in the Conservative Therapy of Patellar Chondropathy," *Beitr. Orthop. Traumatol.*, 1990; 37(5);259-266.

Stenfors, L. E. "Treatment of Tympanic Membrane Perforations with Hyaluronan in an Open Pilot Study of Unselected Patients," *Acta Otolaryngol. (Stockh.)*, 1987; 442 Suppl.:81-87.

Thilo, G. "Untersuchung von 35 Arthrosefallen, Behandelt mit Chondroitinschwefelsaure," *Schweiz. Rundschau Med. (Praxis)*, 1977; 66:1896-1899.

Wiig, M., D. Amiel, and L. Kitabayashi. "Potential Use of Hyaluronan in the Healing of ACL," *Med. Sci. Sports Exer.*, 1988; 20(2)Suppl.:S37.

CHAPTER 6:
ANTIOXIDANTS AGAINST ARTHRITIS

Blankenhorn, G. "Clinical Effectiveness of Spondyvit (vitamin E) in Activated Arthroses. A Multicenter Placebo-Controlled Double Blind Study," *Z. Orthop. Ihre Grenzgeb.*, 1986; 125:340-343.

Biskind, M. A., and W. C. Martin. "The Use of Citrus Flavonoids in Infection. II.", *Am. J. Digest. Dis.*, 1955; 2:41-42.

Bucci, L. R. "Reversal of Osteoarthritis by Nutritional Intervention," *A.C.A. J. Chiropractic*, 1990; 27(11):69-72.

Bucci, L. R. *Nutrition Applied to Injury Rehabilitation and Sports Medicine*, Boca Raton, Florida: CRC Press, 1994.

Burton, G. W., and K. U. Ingold. "ß-Carotene, an Unusual Type of Lipid Anti-Oxidant," *Science*, 1984; 224:569-571.

Deodhar, S. D., R. Sethi, and R. C. Srimal. "Preliminary Study on Antirheumatic Activity of Curcumin (Diferuloyl Methane)," *Indian J. Med. Res.*, 1980; 71:632-635.

Ehrlich, H. P., H. Tarver, and T. K. Hunt. "Inhibitory Effects of Vitamin E on Collagen Synthesis and Wound Repair," *Ann. Surg.*, 1972; 175:235-239.

Greenwood, J. "Optimum Vitamin C Intake as a Factor in the Preservation of Disc Integrity," *Med. Ann. Dist. Columbia*, 1964; 33:274-275.

Halliwell, B., and J. M. C. Gutteridge. *Free Radicals in Biology and Medicine*, 2nd ed., Oxford: Clarendon Press, 1989.

Kamimura, M. "Anti-Inflammatory Effect of Vitamin E," *J. Vitaminol.*, 1972; 18:204-207.

Kienholz, E. W. "Vitamin E, Selenium, and Knee Problems," *Lancet*, 1975; 1:531-532.

Lytle, R. L. "Chronic Dental Pain: Possible Benefits of Food Restriction and Sodium Ascorbate," *J. Appl. Nutr.*, 1988; 40:95-102.

Machtey, I., and L. Ouaknine. "Tocopherol in Osteoarthritis: A Controlled Pilot Study," *J. Am. Ger. Soc.*, 1978; 26:328-330.

Mézes, M., A. Par, G. Bartosiewicz, and J. Nemeth. "Vitamin E Content and Lipid Peroxidation of Blood in Some Chronic Inflammatory Diseases," *Acta Physiol. Hung.*, 1987; 69(1):133-138.

Rubyk, B. I., N. M. Fil'chagin, and R. A. Sabadyshin. "Change in Lipid Peroxidation in Patients with Primary Osteoarthrosis Deformans," *Ter. Arkh.*, 1988; 60:110-115.

Satoskar, R. R., S. J. Shah, and S. G. Shenoy. "Evaluation of Antiinflammatory Property of Curcumin (Diferuloyl Methane) in Patients with Postoperative Inflammation," *Int. J. Clin. Pharmacol. Ther. Toxicol.*, 1986; 24(12):651-653.

Schwartz, E. R. "The Modulation of Osteoarthritic Development by Vitamins C and E," *Int. J. Vit. Nutr. Res.*, 1984; Suppl. 26:141-146.

Schwartz, E. R. "Metabolic Response During Early Stages of Surgically-Induced Osteoarthritis in Mature Beagles," *J. Rheumatol.*, 1980; 7:788-792.

Schwartz, P. L. "Ascorbic Acid in Wound Healing–A Review," *J. Am. Diet. Assoc.*, 1970; 56:497-503.

Sharma, O. P. "Antioxidant Activity of Curcumin and Related Compounds," *Biochem. Pharmacol.*, 1976; 26:1,811-1,818.

Swaak, A. J. G., and J. F. Koster, eds. *Free Radicals and Arthritic Diseases*, Rijswijk, The Netherlands: Eurage, 1986.

CHAPTER 7:
SECOND-LINE NUTRIENTS FOR ARTHRITIS

Abraham, G. E., and H. Grewal. "A Total Dietary Program Emphasizing Magnesium Instead of Calcium. Effect on the Bone Mineral Density of Calcaneous Bone in Postmenopausal Women on Hormonal Therapy," *J. Reprod. Med.*, 1990; 35:503-506.

Anonymous. "Rheumatoid Arthritis and Selenium," *Nutr. Rev.*, 1988; 46:284-286.

Bucci, L. R. "Manganese: Its Role in Nutritional Balance," *Today's Chiropractor*, 1988; 17(2):23-26 and 17(3):45-47.

Bucci, L. R. *Nutrition Applied to Injury Rehabilitation and Sports Medicine*, Boca Raton, Florida: CRC Press, 1994.

Cimmino, M. A., A. Mazzucotelli, G. Rovetta, G. Bianchi, and M. Cutolo. "The Controversy Over Zinc Sulphate Efficacy in Rheumatoid and Psoriatic Arthritis," *Scand. J. Rheumatol.*, 1984; 13:191-192.

Ellis, J. M., and K. Folkers. "Clinical Aspects of Treatment of Carpal Tunnel Syndrome with Vitamin B_6," *Ann. N. Y. Acad. Sci.*, 1990; 585:302-308.

Erasmus, U. *Fats and Oils*, Vancouver: Alive Press, 1987.

Fincham, J. E., S. J. van Rensburg, and W. F. O. Marasas. "Mseleni Joint Disease–A Manganese Deficiency?," *S.A. Med. J.*, 1981; 60(12):445-447.

Hill, J., and H. A. Bird. "Failure of Selenium-ACE to Improve Osteoarthritis," *Br. J. Rheumatol.*, 1990; 29:211-213.

Hoffer, A. "Treatment of Arthritis by Nicotinic Acid and Nicotinamide," *Can. Med. Assoc. J.*, 1959; 81:235-238.

Jameson, S. "Pain Relief and Selenium Balance in Patients with Connective Tissue Disease and Osteoarthrosis: A Double-Blind Selenium Tocopherol Supplementation Study," *Nutr. Res.*, 1985; Suppl. 1:391-396.

Jiang, Y. F., and G. L. Xu. "The Relativity Between Some Epidemiological Characteristics of Kaschin-Beck Disease and Selenium Deficiency," in *Selenium in Biology and Medicine*, Wendel. A., Ed., Berlin: Springer-Verlag, 1988, 263-269.

Kaufman, W. *The Common Form of Joint Dysfunction: Its Incidence and Treatment*, Brattleboro, Vermont: E. L. Hildreth, 1949.

Kaufman, W. "Niacinamide Therapy for Joint Mobility," *Conn. Med. J.*, 1953; 17:584-587.

Kaufman, W. "The Use of Vitamin Therapy to Reverse Certain Concomitants of Aging," *J. Am. Ger. Soc.*, 1955; 3:927-936.

Kaufman, W. "Niacinamide: A Most Neglected Vitamin," *J. Int. Acad. Prev. Med.*, 1983; 8, 5-25.

Newnham, R. E. "Mineral Imbalance and Boron Deficiency," in *Trace Element Metabolism in Man and Animals*, J. M. Gawthorne, J. M. Howell, C. L. White, eds., Berlin: Springer-Verlag, 1982, 400-402.

Newnham, R. E. "The Role of Boron in Human and Animal Health," in *Trace Elements in Man and Animals 7*, B. Momcilovic, Ed., Zagreb: IMI, 1991, 8.4.

Nielsen, F. H., C. D. Hunt , L. M. Mullen, and J. R. Hunt. "Effect of Dietary Boron on Mineral, Estrogen, and Testosterone Metabolism in Postmenopausal Women," *FASEB J.*, 1987; 1:394-397.

Nielsen, F. H. "Facts and Fallacies About Boron," *Nutr. Today*, 1992; May/Jun:6-12.

Nielsen, F. H. "Ultratrace Elements of Possible Importance for Human Health: An Update," in *Essential and Toxic Trace Elements in Human Health and Disease: An Update*, A. S. Prasad, Ed., New York: Wiley-Liss, 1993, 355-367.

Pennington, J. A. T., B. E. Young, D. B. Wilson, R. D. Johnson, and J. E. Vanderveen. "Mineral Content of Foods and Total Diets: The Selected Minerals in Foods Survey, 1982 to 1984," *J. Am. Diet. Assoc.*, 1986; 86:876-891.

Rudin, D. O., and C. Felix. *The Omega-3 Phenomenon*, New York: Rawson Associates, 1987.

Schor, R.A., S. G. Prussin, D. L. Jewett, J. J. Ludowieg, and R. S. Bhatnagar. "Trace levels of manganese, copper, and zinc in rib cartilage as related to age in humans and animals, both normal and dwarfed," *Clin. Orthop.*, 1973; 93:346-353.

Sorenson, J. R. J. "Antiarthritic, Antiulcer, and Analgesic Activities of Copper Complexes," in *Trace Elements in Clinical Medicine*, H. Tomita, Ed., Tokyo: Springer-Verlag, 1990, 261-283.

Travers, R. L., and G. C. Rennie. "Clinical Trial - Boron and Arthritis," *Townsend Lett.*, 1990; 83:360-362.

Walker, W. R. "The Results of a Copper Bracelet Clinical Trial and Subsequent Studies," in *Inflammatory Diseases and Copper*, J. R. J. Sorenson, Ed., Clifton, New Jersey: Humana Press, 1982, 469-481.

CHAPTER 8:
SUPPLEMENTS THAT ACCELERATE HEALING

Baumuller, M. "Therapy of Ankle Joint Distortions with Hydrolytic Enzymes–Results From a Double Blind Clinical Trial," in *Sports, Medicine and Health*, G. P. H. Hermans, W. L. Mosterd, eds., Amsterdam: Excerpta Medica, 1990, 1,137-1,139.

Blonstein, J. L. "Oral Enzyme Tablets in the Treatment of Boxing Injuries," *Practitioner*, 1967; 198:547-548.

Bucci, L. R., and J. C. Stiles. "Sport Injuries and Proteolytic Enzymes," *Today's Chiropractor*, 1987; 16(1):31-34.

Bucci, L. R. "Normal Cellular Components: Proteases, Nucleic Acids and Antioxidant Enzymes," Chapter 11, in *Nutrition Applied to Injury Rehabilitation and Sports Medicine*, Boca Raton, Florida: CRC Press, 1994.

Christie, R. B. "The Medical Uses of Proteolytic Enzymes," in *Topics in Enzyme and Fermentation Biotechnology*, Vol. 4, A. Wiseman, Ed., Chichester, United Kingdom: Ellis Horwood Ltd., 1980, 25-110.

Dietrich, R. E. "Oral Proteolytic Enzymes in the Treatment of Athletic Injuries: A Double-Blind Study," *Penn. Med. J.*, 1965; 68:35-37.

Donaho, C. R., and C. R. Rylander. "Proteolytic Enzymes in Athletic Injuries. A Double-Blind Study of a New Anti-Inflammatory Agent," *Del. Med. J.*, 1962; 34(6):168-170.

Gaspardy, G., G. Balint, M. Mitusova, and G. Lorincz. "Treatment of Sciatica Due to Invertebral Disc Herniation with Chymoral Tablets," *Rheum. Phys. Med.*, 1971; 11:14-17.

Gibson, T., T. F. W. Dilke, and R. Grahame. "Chymoral in the Treatment of Lumbar Disc Prolapse," *Rheum. Rehab.*, 1975; 14:186-189.

Hingorani, K. "Oral Enzyme Therapy in Severe Back Pain," *Br. J. Clin. Prac.*, 1968; 22(5):209-212.

Rahn, H. D. "Efficacy of Hydrolytic Enzymes in Surgery," in *Sports, Medicine and Health*, G. P. H. Hermans, W. L. Mosterd, eds., Amsterdam: Excerpta Medica, 1990, 1,135-1,136.

Trickett, P. "Proteolytic Enzymes in Treatment of Athletic Injuries," *Appl. Ther.*, 1964; 6:647-654.

PART III

CHAPTER 9:
DIETARY SUPPORT FOR YOUR JOINTS

Bucci, L. R. "Nutrients Applied to Injury Rehabilitation and Sports Medicine," Chapter 14 in *Nutrition Applied to Injury Rehabilitation and Sports Medicine*, Boca Raton, Florida: CRC Press, 1994, 215-224.

Brandt, K. D. and H. J. Mankin. "Pathogenesis of Osteoarthritis," Chapter 24 in *Arthritis Surgery*, C. B. Sledge, S. Ruddy, S. D. Harris, W. N. Kelley, eds. Philadelphia: W. B. Saunders, 1994, 450-468.

Erasmus, U. *Fats and Oils*, Vancouver: Alive Press, 1987.

Pennington, J. A. T. *Bowe's and Church's Food Values of Portions Commonly Used*, 15th Ed., Philadelphia: J. B. Lippincott, 1989.

Rudin, D. O., and C. Felix. *The Omega-3 Phenomenon*, New York: Rawson Associates, 1987.

Strickland, E. H., and D. R. Davis, NutriCircles Dietary Analysis Program, Strickland Computing Company, P.O. Box 1255, Valley Center, California, 92082.

CHAPTER 10:
NUTRITIONAL DEFENSE AGAINST SPECIFIC JOINT PROBLEMS

American Academy of Orthopaedic Surgeons, *Athletic Training and Sports Medicine*, 2nd ed., Park Ridge, Illinois: American Academy of Orthopaedic Surgeons, 1991.

Bucci, L. R. "Nutrients Applied to Injury Rehabilitation and Sports Medicine," Chapter 14 in *Nutrition Applied to Injury Rehabilitation and Sports Medicine*, Boca Raton, Florida: CRC Press, 1994, 215-224.

Emery, S. E., H. H. Bohlman. "Osteoarthritis of the Cervical Spine," Chapter 30 in *Osteoarthritis. Diagnosis and Medical/Surgical Management*, 2nd ed., R. W. Moskowitz, D. S. Howell, V. M. Goldberg, H. J. Mankin, eds., Philadelphia: W. B. Saunders, 1992, 651-668.

Figgie, M. P., H. E. Figgie, V. M. Goldberg, and A. E. Inglis. "Osteoarthritis of the Elbow and Shoulder," Chapter 26 in *Osteoarthritis. Diagnosis and Medical/Surgical Management*, 2nd ed., R. W. Moskowitz, D. S. Howell, V. M. Goldberg, H. J. Mankin, eds., Philadelphia: W. B. Saunders, 1992, 561-578.

Frymoyer, J. W., R. E. Booth, and R. H. Rothman. "Osteoarthritis Syndromes of the Lumbar Spine," Chapter 32 in *Osteoarthritis. Diagnosis and Medical/Surgical Management*, 2nd ed., R. W. Moskowitz, D. S. Howell, V. M. Goldberg, H. J. Mankin, eds., Philadelphia: W. B. Saunders, 1992, 683-736.

Gamble, J. G. *The Musculoskeletal System. Physiological Basics*, New York: Raven, 1988.

Goldberg, V. M., D. B. Kettelkamp, and R. A. Colyer. "Osteoarthritis of the Knee," Chapter 28 in *Osteoarthritis. Diagnosis and Medical/Surgical Management*, 2nd ed., R. W. Moskowitz, D. S. Howell, V. M. Goldberg, H. J. Mankin, eds., Philadelphia: W. B. Saunders, 1992, 599-620.

Gould, J. S. "Painful Feet," Chapter 91 in *Arthritis and Allied Conditions. A Textbook of Rheumatology*, Vol. 2, 12th ed., D. J. McCarty, W. J. Koopman, eds., Philadelphia: Lea and Febiger, 1993, 1,553-1,561.

Hardin, J.G., J. T. Halla. "Cervical Spine Syndromes," Chapter 92 in *Arthritis and Allied Conditions. A Textbook of Rheumatology*, Vol. 2, 12th ed., D. J. McCarty, W. J. Koopman, eds., Philadelphia: Lea and Febiger, 1993, 1,563-1,571.

Hardy, R. W. "Osteoarthritis of the Thoracic Spine," Chapter 31 in *Osteoarthritis. Diagnosis and Medical/Surgical Management*, 2nd ed., R. W. Moskowitz, D. S. Howell, V. M. Goldberg, H. J. Mankin, eds., Philadelphia: W. B. Saunders, 1992, 669-681.

Levine, D. B., and J. M. Leipzig. "The Painful Back," Chapter 94 in *Arthritis and Allied Conditions. A Textbook of Rheumatology*, Vol. 2, 12th ed., D. J. McCarty, W. J. Koopman, eds., Philadelphia: Lea and Febiger, 1993, 1,583-1,600.

Lipson, S. J. "Low Back Pain," Chapter 15 in *Arthritis Surgery*, C. B. Sledge, S. Ruddy, E. D. Harris, W. N. Kelley, eds., Philadelphia: W. B. Saunders, 1994, 225-242.

Mann, R. A. "Osteoarthritis of the Foot and Ankle," Chapter 27 in *Osteoarthritis. Diagnosis and Medical/Surgical Management*, 2nd ed., R. W. Moskowitz, D. S. Howell, V. M. Goldberg, H. J. Mankin, eds., Philadelphia: W. B. Saunders, 1992, 579-598.

McCarty, D. J., and W. J. Koopman, eds., *Arthritis and Allied Conditions. A Textbook of Rheumatology*. Vol. 2, 12th ed., Philadelphia: Lea and Febiger, 1993.

McLatchie, G. R., C. M. E. Lennox, E. C. Percy, and J. Davies., eds., *The Soft Tissues. Trauma and Sports Injuries*, Oxford: Butterworth-Heinemann, 1993.

Moskowitz, R. W. "Osteoarthritis–Symptoms and Signs," Chapter 10 in *Osteoarthritis. Diagnosis and Medical/Surgical Management*, 2nd ed., R. W. Moskowitz, D. S. Howell, V. M. Goldberg, H. J. Mankin, eds., Philadelphia: W. B. Saunders, 1992, 255-261.

Nakano, K. K. "Neck Pain," Chapter 13 in *Arthritis Surgery*, C. B. Sledge, S. Ruddy, E. D. Harris, W. N. Kelley, eds., Philadelphia: W. B. Saunders, 1994, 225-242.

Norris, C. M. *Sports Injuries. Diagnosis and Management for Physiotherapists*, Oxford: Butterworth-Heinemann, 1993.

O'Duffy, J. D., and M. J. Ebersold. "Spinal Stenosis," Chapter 95 in *Arthritis and Allied Conditions. A Textbook of Rheumatology*, Vol. 2, 12th ed., D. J. McCarty, W. J. Koopman, eds., Philadelphia: Lea and Febiger, 1993, 1,601-1,608.

Parks, R. M. "Lower Extremity Sports Injuries," Chapter 5 in *Sports and Exercise Medicine*, S. C. Wood, R. C. Roach, eds., New York: Marcel Dekker, 1994.

Poland, J. L., D. J. Hobart, and O. D. Payton, *The Musculoskeletal System*, 2nd. ed., Garden City, New York: Medical Examination Publishing, 1981.

Renström, P. A. F. H., Ed., *Sports Injuries. Basic Principles of Prevention and Care*, Oxford: Blackwell Scientific Publications, 1993.

Rosse, C., and D. K. Clawson, eds. *The Musculoskeletal System in Health and Disease*, Hagerstown, Pennsylvania: Harper and Row, 1980.

Ryan, D. E. "Painful Temporomandibular Joint." Chapter 93 in *Arthritis and Allied Conditions. A Textbook of Rheumatology*, Vol. 2, 12th ed., D. J. McCarty, W. J. Koopman, eds., Philadelphia: Lea and Febiger, 1993, 1,573-1,582.

Siegel, D. B., R. H. Gelberman, and R. Smith. "Osteoarthritis of the Hand and Wrist," Chapter 25 in *Osteoarthritis. Diagnosis and Medical/Surgical Management*, 2nd ed., R. W. Moskowitz, D. S. Howell, V. M. Goldberg, H. J. Mankin, eds., Philadelphia: W. B. Saunders, 1992, 547-559.

Staufer, R. N. "Correction of Arthritic Deformities of the Hip," Chapter 53 in *Arthritis and Allied Conditions. A Textbook of Rheumatology*, Vol. 1, 12th ed., D. J. McCarty, W. J. Koopman, eds., Philadelphia: Lea and Febiger, 1993, 969-980.

Thornhill, T. S. "Shoulder Pain," Chapter 14 in *Arthritis Surgery*, C. B. Sledge, S. Ruddy, E. D. Harris, W. N. Kelley, eds., Philadelphia: W. B. Saunders, 1994, 201-224.

Tsahakis, P. J., G. W. Brick, and R. Poss. "Surgery of the Hip," Chapter 43 in *Arthritis Surgery*, C. B. Sledge, S. Ruddy, E. D. Harris, W. N. Kelley, eds., Philadelphia: W. B. Saunders, 1994, 780-793.

Wilson, M. G., and R. Poss R. "Osteoarthritis of the Hip," Chapter 29 in *Osteoarthritis. Diagnosis and Medical/Surgical Management*, 2nd ed., R. W. Moskowitz, D. S. Howell, V. M. Goldberg, H. J. Mankin, eds., Philadelphia: W. B. Saunders, 1992, 621-649.

CHAPTER 11:
RATING THE ARTHRITIS DRUGS

Altman, R. D., P. Kapila, D. D. Dean, and D. S. Howell. "Future Therapeutic Trends in Osteoarthritis," *Scand. J. Rheumatol. Suppl.*, 1988; 77:37-42.

American Academy of Orthopaedic Surgeons, "Rehabilitative Techniques," Section Six in *Athletic Training and Sports Medicine*, 2nd ed., Park Ridge, Illinois: American Academy of Orthopaedic Surgeons, 1991, 773-846.

Arsenis, C., and J. McDonnell. "Effects of Antirheumatic Drugs on the Interleukin-1 Alpha Induced Synthesis and Activation of Proteinases in Articular Cartilage Explants in Culture," *Agents-Actions*, 1989; 27:261-264.

Batchlor, E. E., and H. E. Paulus. "Principles of Drug Therapy," Chapter 20 in *Osteoarthritis. Diagnosis and Medical/Surgical Management*, 2nd ed., R. W. Moskowitz, D. S. Howell, V. M. Goldberg, H. J. Mankin, eds., Philadelphia: W. B. Saunders, 1992, 465-492.

Bird, H. "The Current Treatment of Osteoarthritis," Chapter 17 in *Osteoarthritis. Current Research and Prospects for Pharmacological Intervention*, R. G. G. Russell, P. A. Dieppe, eds., London: IBC Technical Services Ltd., 1991, 173-196.

Bjelle, A., and I. Eronen. "The In Vitro Effect of Six NSAIDs on the Glycosaminoglycan Metabolism of Rabbit Chondrocytes," *Clin. Exp. Rheumatol.*, 1991; 9:369-374.

Brandt, K. "Drug-Induced Changes in Cartilage. Do NSAIDs. Influence the Outcome of Degenerative Joint Disease?," in *Degenerative Joints*, Vol. 2, G. Verbruggen, E. M. Veys, eds., Amsterdam: Excerpta Medica, 1985, 315-323.

Brandt, K. D. "Nonsteroidal Antiinflammatory Drugs and Articular Cartilage," *J. Rheumatol.*, 1987; Suppl. 14:132-133.

Brandt, K. D., and D. Flusser. "Osteoarthritis," Chapter 2 in *Prognosis in the Rheumatic Diseases*, N. Bellamy, Ed., Dordrecht, Germany: Kluwer Academic Publishers, 1991, 11-36.

Curl, W. W., and D. F. Martin. "Initial Management of Acute Injuries," Chapter 34 in *Sports Injuries. Basic Principles of Prevention and Care*, Renström P. A. F. H., Ed., Oxford: Blackwell Scientific Publications, 1993, 437-448.

David, M. J., E. Vignon, M. J. Peschard, P. Broquet, P. Louisot, and M. Richard. "Effect of Non-Steroidal Anti-Inflammatory Drugs (NSAID.S.) on Glycosyltransferase Activity from Human Osteoarthritic Cartilage," *Br. J. Rheumatol.*, 1992; 31 (Suppl. 1):13-17.

de Vries, B. J., P. M. van der Kraan, W. B. van den Berg. "Decrease of Inorganic Blood Sulfate Following Treatment with Selected Antirheumatic Drugs: Potential Consequences for Articular Cartilage," *Agents-Actions*, 1990; 29:224-231.

Dingle, J. T. "Prostaglandins in Human Cartilage Metabolism," *J. Lipid Mediat.*, 1993, 6:303-312.

Emery, S. E., and H. H. Bohlman. "Osteoarthritis of the Cervical Spine," Chapter 30 in *Osteoarthritis. Diagnosis and Medical/Surgical Management*, 2nd ed., R. W. Moskowitz, D. S. Howell, V. M. Goldberg, H. J. Mankin, eds., Philadelphia: W. B. Saunders, 1992, 651-668.

Fife, R.S., and K. D. Brandt. "Other Approaches to Therapy," Chapter 22 in *Osteoarthritis. Diagnosis and Medical/Surgical Management*, 2nd ed., R. W. Moskowitz, D. S. Howell, V. M. Goldberg, H. J. Mankin, eds., Philadelphia: W. B. Saunders, 1992, 511-526.

Figgie, M. P., H. E. Figgie, V. M. Goldberg, and A. E. Inglis. "Osteoarthritis of the Elbow and Shoulder," Chapter 26 in *Osteoarthritis. Diagnosis and Medical/Surgical Management*, 2nd ed., R. W. Moskowitz, D. S. Howell, V. M. Goldberg, H. J. Mankin, eds., Philadelphia: W. B. Saunders, 1992, 561-578.

Frymoyer, J. W., R. E. Booth, and R. H. Rothman. "Osteoarthritis Syndromes of the Lumbar Spine," Chapter 32 in *Osteoarthritis. Diagnosis and Medical/Surgical Management*, 2nd ed., R. W. Moskowitz, D. S. Howell, V. M. Goldberg, H. J. Mankin, eds., Philadelphia: W. B. Saunders, 1992, 683-736.

Ghosh, P. "Anti-Rheumatic Drugs and Cartilage," *Baillieres Clin. Rheumatol.*, 1988; 2(2):309-338.

Goldberg, V. M. "Surgery in Osteoarthritis: General Considerations," Chapter 24 in *Osteoarthritis. Diagnosis and Medical/Surgical Management,* 2nd ed., R. W. Moskowitz, D. S. Howell, V. M. Goldberg, H. J. Mankin, eds., Philadelphia: W. B. Saunders, 1992, 535-544.

Goldberg, V. M., D. B. Kettelkamp, and R. A. Colyer. "Osteoarthritis of the Knee," Chapter 28 in *Osteoarthritis. Diagnosis and Medical/Surgical Management,* 2nd ed., R. W. Moskowitz, D. S. Howell, V. M. Goldberg, H. J. Mankin, eds., Philadelphia: W. B. Saunders, 1992, 599-620.

Gould, J. S. "Painful Feet," Chapter 91 in *Arthritis and Allied Conditions. A Textbook of Rheumatology,* Vol. 2, 12th ed., D. J. McCarty, W. J. Koopman, eds., Philadelphia: Lea and Febiger, 1993, 1,553-1,561.

Hardin, J.G., and J. T. Halla. "Cervical Spine Syndromes," Chapter 92 in *Arthritis and Allied Conditions. A Textbook of Rheumatology,* Vol. 2, 12th ed., D. J. McCarty, W. J. Koopman, eds., Philadelphia: Lea and Febiger, 1993, 1,563-1,571.

Hardy, R. W. "Osteoarthritis of the Thoracic Spine," Chapter 31 in *Osteoarthritis. Diagnosis and Medical/Surgical Management,* 2nd ed., R. W. Moskowitz, D. S. Howell, V. M. Goldberg, H. J. Mankin, eds., Philadelphia: W. B. Saunders, 1992, 669-681.

Herman, J. H., A. M. Appel, R. C. Khosla, and E. V. Hess. "The *In Vitro* effect of Select Classes of Nonsteroidal Anti-inflammatory Drugs on Normal Cartilage Metabolism," *J. Rheumatol.,* 1986; 13:1,014-1,018.

Hicks, J. E., and L. H. Gerber. "Rehabilitation on the Management of Patients with Osteoarthritis," Chapter 19 in *Osteoarthritis. Diagnosis and Medical/Surgical Management,* 2nd ed., R. W. Moskowitz, D. S. Howell, V. M. Goldberg, H. J. Mankin, eds., Philadelphia: W. B. Saunders, 1992, 427-464.

Jackson, R. W. "The Role of Arthroscopy in Diagnosis and Management of Osteoarthritis," Chapter 23 in *Osteoarthritis. Diagnosis and Medical/Surgical Management,* 2nd ed., R. W. Moskowitz, D. S. Howell, V. M. Goldberg, H. J. Mankin, eds., Philadelphia: W. B. Saunders, 1992, 527-534.

Kalbhen, D. A. "Degenerative Joint Disease Following Chondrocyte Injury— Chemically Induced Osteoarthritis," in *Degenerative Joints,* Vol. 2, G. Verbruggen, E. M. Veys, eds., Amsterdam: Excerpta Medica, 1985, 299-313.

Kalbhen, D. A. "The Influence of NSAIDs on Morphology of Articular Cartilage," *Scand. J. Rheumatol. Suppl.,* 1988; 77:13-22.

Levine, D. B., and J. M. Leipzig. "The Painful Back," Chapter 94 in *Arthritis and Allied Conditions. A Textbook of Rheumatology,* Vol. 2, 12th ed., D. J. McCarty, W. J. Koopman, eds., Philadelphia: Lea and Febiger, 1993, 1,583-1,600.

Lipson, S. J. "Low Back Pain," Chapter 15 in *Arthritis Surgery,* C. B. Sledge, S. Ruddy, E. D. Harris, W. N. Kelley, eds., Philadelphia: W. B. Saunders, 1994, 225-242.

Mann, R. A. "Osteoarthritis of the Foot and Ankle," Chapter 27 in *Osteoarthritis. Diagnosis and Medical/Surgical Management,* 2nd ed., R. W. Moskowitz, D. S. Howell, V. M. Goldberg, H. J. Mankin, eds., Philadelphia: W. B. Saunders, 1992, 579-598.

Morrey, B. F. "Surgery of the Elbow," Chapter 40 in *Arthritis Surgery,* C. B. Sledge, S. Ruddy, E. D. Harris, W. N. Kelley, eds., Philadelphia: W. B. Saunders, 1994, 733-753.

Moskowitz, R. W. "Osteoarthritis–Symptoms and Signs," Chapter 10 in *Osteoarthritis. Diagnosis and Medical/Surgical Management,* 2nd ed., R. W. Moskowitz, D. S. Howell, V. M. Goldberg, H. J. Mankin, eds., Philadelphia: W. B. Saunders, 1992, 255-261.

Nakano, K. K. "Neck Pain," Chapter 13 in *Arthritis Surgery,* C. B. Sledge, S. Ruddy, E. D. Harris, W. N. Kelley, eds., Philadelphia: W. B. Saunders, 1994, 225-242.

Neer, C. S. "Surgery of the Shoulder," Chapter 41 in *Arthritis Surgery*, C. B. Sledge, S. Ruddy, E. D. Harris, W. N. Kelley, eds., Philadelphia: W. B. Saunders, 1994, 754-769.

Neustadt, D. H. "Intra-Articular Steroid Therapy," Chapter 21 in *Osteoarthritis. Diagnosis and Medical/Surgical Management*, 2nd ed., R. W. Moskowitz, D. S. Howell, V. M. Goldberg, H. J. Mankin, eds., Philadelphia: W. B. Saunders, 1992, 493-510.

Newman, N. M., and R. S. M. Ling. "Acetabular Bone Destruction Related to Non-Steroidal Anti-Inflammatory Drugs," *Lancet*, 1985; 2:11-14.

Norris, C. M. "Part Two," Chapters 9-22 in *Sports Injuries. Diagnosis and Management for Physiotherapists*, Oxford: Butterworth-Heinemann, 1993, 147-315.

Obeid, G., X. Zhang, and X. Wang. "Effect of Ibuprofen on the Healing and Remodeling of Bone and Articular Cartilage in the Rabbit Temporomandibular Joint," *J. Oral Maxillofac. Surg.*, 1992; 50:843-849.

O'Duffy, J. D., and M. J. Ebersold. "Spinal Stenosis," Chapter 95 in *Arthritis and Allied Conditions. A Textbook of Rheumatology*, Vol. 2, 12th ed., D. J. McCarty, W. J. Koopman, eds., Philadelphia: Lea and Febiger, 1993, 1,601-1,608.

Paulos, L., and M. Kody. "Management of the Acutely Injured Joint," Chapter 5 in *The Soft Tissues. Trauma and Sports Injuries*, G. R. McLatchie, C. M. E. Lennox, E. C. Percy, and J. Davies, eds., Oxford: Butterworth-Heinemann, 1993, 104-124.

Pelletier, J. P., J. M. Cliutier, and J. Martel-Pelletier. "*In Vitro* Effects of Tiaprofenic Acid, Sodium Salicylate and Hydrocortisone on the Proteoglycan Metabolism of Human Osteoarthritic Cartilage," *J. Rheumatol.*, 1989; 16:646-655.

Rashad, S., P. Revell, A. Hemingway, F. Low, K. Rainsford, and F. Walker. "Effect of Nonsteroidal Anti-Inflammatory Drugs on the Course of Osteoarthritis," *Lancet*, 1989; 2:519-522.

Ronningen, H., and N. Langeland. "Indomethacin Hips," *Acta Orthop. Scand.*, 1977; 48:556.

Ryan, D. E. "Painful Temporomandibular Joint," Chapter 93 in *Arthritis and Allied Conditions. A Textbook of Rheumatology*, Vol. 2, 12th ed., D. J. McCarty, W. J. Koopman, eds., Philadelphia: Lea and Febiger, 1993, 1,573-1,582.

Saltzman, C. L., and K. A. Johnson. "Surgery of the Ankle and Foot," Chapter 45 in *Arthritis and Allied Conditions. A Textbook of Rheumatology*, Vol. 1, 12th ed., D. J. McCarty, W. J. Koopman, eds., Philadelphia: Lea and Febiger, 1993, 818-837.

Schnitzer, T. J. "Management of Osteoarthritis," Chapter 104 in *Arthritis and Allied Conditions. A Textbook of Rheumatology*, Vol. 2, 12th ed., D. J. McCarty, W. J. Koopman, eds., Philadelphia: Lea and Febiger, 1993, 1,761-1,769

Siegel, D. B., R. H. Gelberman, and R. Smith. "Osteoarthritis of the Hand and Wrist," Chapter 25 in *Osteoarthritis. Diagnosis and Medical/Surgical Management*, 2nd ed., R. W. Moskowitz, D. S. Howell, V. M. Goldberg, H. J. Mankin, eds., Philadelphia: W. B. Saunders, 1992, 547-559.

Simmons, B. P., L. H. Millender, and E. A. Nalebuff. "Surgery of the Hand," Chapter 39 in *Arthritis and Allied Conditions. A Textbook of Rheumatology*, Vol. 1, 12th ed., D. J. McCarty, W. J. Koopman, eds., Philadelphia: Lea and Febiger, 1993, 706-732.

Soren, A. *Arthritis and Related Affections. Clinic, Pathology, and Treatment*, Berlin: Springer-Verlag, 1993, 205-238.

Staufer, R. N. "Correction of Arthritic Deformities of the Hip," Chapter 53 in *Arthritis and Allied Conditions. A Textbook of Rheumatology*, Vol. 1, 12th ed., D. J. McCarty, W. J. Koopman, eds., Philadelphia: Lea and Febiger, 1993, 969-980.

Thornhill, T. S. "Shoulder Pain," Chapter 14 in *Arthritis Surgery*, C. B. Sledge, S. Ruddy, E. D. Harris, W. N. Kelley, eds., Philadelphia: W. B. Saunders, 1994, 201-224.

Tsahakis, P. J., G. W. Brick, and R. Poss. "Surgery of the Hip," Chapter 43 in *Arthritis Surgery*, C. B. Sledge, S. Ruddy, E. D. Harris, W. N. Kelley, eds., Philadelphia: W. B. Saunders, 1994, 780-793.

Wilson, M. G., and R. Poss. "Osteoarthritis of the Hip," Chapter 29 in *Osteoarthritis. Diagnosis and Medical/Surgical Management*, 2nd ed., R. W. Moskowitz, D. S. Howell, V. M. Goldberg, H. J. Mankin, eds., Philadelphia: W. B. Saunders, 1992, 621-649.

Windsor, R. E., J. N. Insall. "Surgery of the Knee," Chapter 44 in *Arthritis Surgery*, C. B. Sledge, S. Ruddy, E. D. Harris, W. N. Kelley, eds., Philadelphia: W. B. Saunders, 1994, 794-817.

CHAPTER 12:
GOING UNDER THE KNIFE: A REALISTIC OPTION?

American Academy of Orthopaedic Surgeons, Rehabilitative techniques, Section Six in *Athletic Training and Sports Medicine*, 2nd ed., Park Ridge, Illinois: American Academy of Orthopaedic Surgeons, 1991, 773-846.

Emery, S. E., and H. H. Bohlman. "Osteoarthritis of the Cervical Spine," Chapter 30 in *Osteoarthritis. Diagnosis and Medical/Surgical Management*, 2nd ed., R. W. Moskowitz, D. S. Howell, V. M. Goldberg, H. J. Mankin, eds., Philadelphia: W. B. Saunders, 1992, 651-668.

Fife, R. S., and K. D. Brandt. "Other Approaches to Therapy," Chapter 22 in *Osteoarthritis. Diagnosis and Medical/Surgical Management*, 2nd ed., R. W. Moskowitz, D. S. Howell, V. M. Goldberg, H. J. Mankin, eds., Philadelphia: W. B. Saunders, 1992, 511-526.

Figgie, M. P., H. E. Figgie, V. M. Goldberg, and A. E. Inglis. "Osteoarthritis of the Elbow and Shoulder," Chapter 26 in *Osteoarthritis. Diagnosis and Medical/Surgical Management*, 2nd ed., R. W. Moskowitz, D. S. Howell, V. M. Goldberg, H. J. Mankin, eds., Philadelphia: W. B. Saunders, 1992, 561-578.

Frymoyer, J. W., R. E. Booth, and R. H. Rothman. "Osteoarthritis Syndromes of the Lumbar Spine," Chapter 32 in *Osteoarthritis. Diagnosis and Medical/Surgical Management*, 2nd ed., R. W. Moskowitz, D. S. Howell, V. M. Goldberg, H. J. Mankin, eds., Philadelphia: W. B. Saunders, 1992, 683-736.

Goldberg, V. M. "Surgery in Osteoarthritis: General Considerations," Chapter 24 in *Osteoarthritis. Diagnosis and Medical/Surgical Management*, 2nd ed., R. W. Moskowitz, D. S. Howell, V. M. Goldberg, H. J. Mankin, eds., Philadelphia: W. B. Saunders, 1992, 535-544.

Goldberg, V. M., D. B. Kettelkamp, and R. A. Colyer. "Osteoarthritis of the Knee," Chapter 28 in *Osteoarthritis. Diagnosis and Medical/Surgical Management*, 2nd ed., R. W. Moskowitz, D. S. Howell, V. M. Goldberg, H. J. Mankin, eds., Philadelphia: W. B. Saunders, 1992, 599-620.

Gould, J. S. "Painful Feet," Chapter 91 in *Arthritis and Allied Conditions. A Textbook of Rheumatology*, Vol. 2, 12th ed., D. J. McCarty, W. J. Koopman, eds., Philadelphia: Lea and Febiger, 1993, 1,553-1,561.

Hardin, J. G., and J. T. Halla. "Cervical Spine Syndromes," Chapter 92 in *Arthritis and Allied Conditions. A Textbook of Rheumatology*, Vol. 2, 12th ed., D. J. McCarty, W. J. Koopman, eds., Philadelphia: Lea and Febiger, 1993, 1,563-1,571.

Hardy, R. W. "Osteoarthritis of the thoracic spine," Chapter 31 in *Osteoarthritis. Diagnosis and Medical/Surgical Management,* 2nd ed., R. W. Moskowitz, D. S. Howell, V. M. Goldberg, H. J. Mankin, eds., Philadelphia: W. B. Saunders, 1992, 669-681.

Hicks, J. E., and L. H. Gerber. "Rehabilitation on the Management of Patients with Osteoarthritis," Chapter 19 in *Osteoarthritis. Diagnosis and Medical/Surgical Management,* 2nd ed., R. W. Moskowitz, D. S. Howell, V. M. Goldberg, H. J. Mankin, eds., Philadelphia: W. B. Saunders, 1992, 427-464.

Jackson, R. W. "The Role of Arthroscopy in Diagnosis and Management of Osteoarthritis," Chapter 23 in *Osteoarthritis. Diagnosis and Medical/Surgical Management,* 2nd ed., R. W. Moskowitz, D. S. Howell, V. M. Goldberg, H. J. Mankin, eds., Philadelphia: W. B. Saunders, 1992, 527-534.

Levine, D. B., and J. M. Leipzig. "The Painful Back," Chapter 94 in *Arthritis and Allied Conditions. A Textbook of Rheumatology,* Vol. 2, 12th ed., D. J. McCarty, W. J. Koopman, eds., Philadelphia: Lea and Febiger, 1993, 1,583-1,600.

Lipson, S. J. "Low Back Pain," Chapter 15 in *Arthritis Surgery,* C. B. Sledge, S. Ruddy, E. D. Harris, W. N. Kelley, eds., Philadelphia: W. B. Saunders, 1994, 225-242.

Mann, R. A. "Osteoarthritis of the Foot and Ankle," Chapter 27 in *Osteoarthritis. Diagnosis and Medical/Surgical Management,* 2nd ed., R. W. Moskowitz, D. S. Howell, V. M. Goldberg, H. J. Mankin, eds., Philadelphia: W. B. Saunders, 1992, 579-598.

Morrey, B. F. "Surgery of the Elbow," Chapter 40 in *Arthritis Surgery,* C. B. Sledge, S. Ruddy, E. D. Harris, W. N. Kelley, eds., Philadelphia: W. B. Saunders, 1994, 733-753.

Nakano, K. K. "Neck Pain," Chapter 13 in *Arthritis Surgery,* C. B. Sledge, S. Ruddy, E. D. Harris, W. N. Kelley, eds., Philadelphia: W. B. Saunders, 1994, 225-242.

Neer, C. S. "Surgery of the Shoulder," Chapter 41 in *Arthritis Surgery,* C. B. Sledge, S. Ruddy, E. D. Harris, W. N. Kelley, eds., Philadelphia: W. B. Saunders, 1994, 754-769.

Norris, C. M. "Part Two," Chapters 9-22 in *Sports Injuries. Diagnosis and Management for Physiotherapists,* Oxford: Butterworth-Heinemann, 1993, 147-315.

O'Duffy, J. D., and M. J. Ebersold. "Spinal Stenosis," Chapter 95 in *Arthritis and Allied Conditions. A Textbook of Rheumatology,* Vol. 2, 12th ed., D. J. McCarty, W. J. Koopman, eds., Philadelphia: Lea and Febiger, 1993, 1,601-1,608.

Ryan, D. E. "Painful Temporomandibular Joint," Chapter 93 in *Arthritis and Allied Conditions. A Textbook of Rheumatology,* Vol. 2, 12th ed., D. J. McCarty, W. J. Koopman, eds., Philadelphia: Lea and Febiger, 1993, 1,573-1,582.

Saltzman, C. L., and K. A. Johnson. "Surgery of the Ankle and Foot," Chapter 45 in *Arthritis and Allied Conditions. A Textbook of Rheumatology,* Vol. 1, 12th ed., D. J. McCarty, W. J. Koopman, eds., Philadelphia: Lea and Febiger, 1993, 818-837.

Schnitzer, T. J. "Management of Osteoarthritis," Chapter 104 in *Arthritis and Allied Conditions. A Textbook of Rheumatology,* Vol. 2, 12th ed., D. J. McCarty, W. J. Koopman, eds., Philadelphia: Lea and Febiger, 1993, 1,761-1,769

Siegel, D. B., R. H. Gelberman, and R. Smith. "Osteoarthritis of the Hand and Wrist," Chapter 25 in *Osteoarthritis. Diagnosis and Medical/Surgical Management,* 2nd ed., R. W. Moskowitz, D. S. Howell, V. M. Goldberg, H. J. Mankin, eds., Philadelphia: W. B. Saunders, 1992, 547-559.

Simmons, B. P., L. H. Millender, and E. A. Nalebuff. "Surgery of the Hand," Chapter 39 in *Arthritis and Allied Conditions. A Textbook of Rheumatology,* Vol. 1, 12th ed., D. J. McCarty, W. J. Koopman, eds., Philadelphia: Lea and Febiger, 1993, 706-732.

Soren, A. *Arthritis and Related Affections. Clinic, Pathology, and Treatment*, Berlin: Springer-Verlag, 1993, 205-238.

Staufer, R. N. "Correction of Arthritic Deformities of the Hip," Chapter 53 in *Arthritis and Allied Conditions. A Textbook of Rheumatology*, Vol. 1, 12th ed., D. J. McCarty, W. J. Koopman, eds., Philadelphia: Lea and Febiger, 1993, 969-980.

Thornhill, T. S. "Shoulder Pain," Chapter 14 in *Arthritis Surgery*, C. B. Sledge, S. Ruddy, E. D. Harris, W. N. Kelley, eds., Philadelphia: W. B. Saunders, 1994, 201-224.

Tsahakis, P. J., G. W. Brick, and R. Poss. "Surgery of the Hip," Chapter 43 in *Arthritis Surgery*, C. B. Sledge, S. Ruddy, E. D. Harris, W. N. Kelley, eds., Philadelphia: W. B. Saunders, 1994, 780-793.

Wilson, M. G., and R. Poss. "Osteoarthritis of the Hip," Chapter 29 in *Osteoarthritis. Diagnosis and Medical/Surgical Management*, 2nd ed., R. W. Moskowitz, D. S. Howell, V. M. Goldberg, H. J. Mankin, eds., Philadelphia: W. B. Saunders, 1992, 621-649.

Windsor, R. E., and J. N. Insall. "Surgery of the Knee," Chapter 44 in *Arthritis Surgery*, C. B. Sledge, S. Ruddy, E. D. Harris, W. N. Kelley, eds., Philadelphia: W. B. Saunders, 1994, 794-817.

CHAPTER 13:
OTHER ARTHRITIS-CARE PROGRAMS: HOW WELL DO THEY WORK?

Altman, R. D., P. Kapila, D. D. Dean, and D. S. Howell. "Future Therapeutic Trends in Osteoarthritis," *Scand. J. Rheumatol. Suppl.*, 1988; 77:37-42.

American Academy of Orthopaedic Surgeons, "Rehabilitative Techniques," Section Six in *Athletic Training and Sports Medicine*, 2nd ed., Park Ridge, Illinois: American Academy of Orthopaedic Surgeons, 1991, 773-846.

Bird, H. "The Current Treatment of Osteoarthritis," Chapter 17 in *Osteoarthritis. Current Research and Prospects for Pharmacological Intervention*, R. G. G. Russell, P. A. Dieppe, eds., London: IBC Technical Services Ltd., 1991, 173-196.

Fife, R. S., and K. D. Brandt. "Other Approaches to Therapy," Chapter 22 in *Osteoarthritis. Diagnosis and Medical/Surgical Management*, 2nd ed., R. W. Moskowitz, D. S. Howell, V. M. Goldberg, H. J. Mankin, eds., Philadelphia: W. B. Saunders, 1992, 511-526.

Hicks, J. E., and L. H. Gerber. "Rehabilitation on the Management of Patients with Osteoarthritis," Chapter 19 in *Osteoarthritis. Diagnosis and Medical/Surgical Management*, 2nd ed., R. W. Moskowitz, D. S. Howell, V. M. Goldberg, H. J. Mankin, eds., Philadelphia: W. B. Saunders, 1992, 427-464.

Norris, C. M. "Part Two," Chapters 9-22 in *Sports Injuries. Diagnosis and Management for Physiotherapists*, Oxford: Butterworth-Heinemann, 1993, 147-315.

Schnitzer, T. J. "Management of Osteoarthritis," Chapter 104 in *Arthritis and Allied Conditions. A Textbook of Rheumatology*, Vol. 2, 12th ed., D. J. McCarty, W. J. Koopman, eds., Philadelphia: Lea and Febiger, 1993, 1,761-1,769

Soren, A. *Arthritis and Related Affections. Clinic, Pathology, and Treatment*, Berlin: Springer-Verlag, 1993, 205-238.

Index

D

E

F

N

O

R

S

W

X

Z